The illnesses caused by tainted food can—and do—kill. Those who don't die may suffer lifelong health problems, ranging from brain damage to breathing, stomach, and heart problems. If you think you're not at risk, think again. The food you eat may host a range of contaminants, including *Salmonella*, *Campylobacter*, *Yersinia*, *Cryptosporidium*, *Listeria*, or the deadly *E. coli* 0157:H7, together with pesticides, viruses, and an accumulation of chemicals and heavy metals. Those at highest risk are children under age sixteen and everybody over sixty.

There *is* plenty you can do to protect yourself—but first you have to know how. . . .

PROTECT YOURSELF FROM CONTAMINATED FOOD AND DRINK

Carol A. Turkington

BALLANTINE BOOKS • NEW YORK

A Ballantine Book
Published by The Ballantine Publishing Group
Copyright © 1999 by Carol A. Turkington

www.randomhouse.com/BB/

Library of Congress Catalog Card Number: 98-96654

ISBN 0-345-42898-6

Manufactured in the United States of America

First Edition: January 1999

10   9   8   7   6   5   4   3   2   1

Contents

Introduction

Every second, ten Americans get sick from food or beverages contaminated with *Salmonella*, *Campylobacter jejuni*, *Yersinia*, *Cryptosporidium*, *Anisakis*, *Listeria*, or *E. coli* 0157:H7, according to the Centers for Disease Control and Prevention.

Every day, twenty-four of them will die.

Yet even as the risk of contamination skyrockets, far too many Americans remain blithely unaware of the problem. Because outbreaks often are not widely reported, most Americans are completely uninformed about the true dimensions of the danger. Consider the following incidents, all of which have occurred in the last few years:

Los Angeles, California, and Milwaukee, Wisconsin 10,000 children and their teachers must be innoculated against hepatitis A after eating contaminated strawberries from Mexico.

Milwaukee, Wisconsin 370,000 residents (one-fourth

of the total population) get sick with cryptosporidiosis from tainted drinking water; 4,000 are hospitalized and several die.

Seattle, Washington 4 die and 700 get sick with deadly
E. coli 0157:H7 poisoning from tainted burgers at a
Jack-in-the-Box restaurant.

Bennington, Vermont 3,000 people are sickened by
water tainted with *Campylobacter jejuni*.

California 150 people get sick and 30 die from *Listeria*-
contaminated cheese.

Central Colorado 94 people contract *Salmonella*-
related hepatitis at a fast-food restaurant.

Carroll County, Georgia 13,000 people get sick after
drinking *Cryptosporidium*-tainted water.

King County, Washington 20 people get sick from
eating dry salami contaminated with *E coli*; 3 are
hospitalized.

Jackson County, Oregon 15,000 people get sick after
drinking tainted water.

Central Maine A wave of students develop cryptosporidiosis after drinking tainted apple cider at an
agricultural fair.

U.S. Northwest and Canada More than 400 men,
women, and children get sick from eating unwashed
Salmonella-contaminated cantaloupe.

Philadelphia, Pennsylvania Citizens are asked to boil
their water because it is contaminated with *Cryptosporidium*.

Orlando, Florida Officials discover a huge plume of
contaminated groundwater with trichloroethylene
levels 40,000 times higher than federal regulations
allow.

New York, New York Officials debate whether to have citizens boil drinking water to protect against contamination.

Washington, D.C. Entire population must boil water for five days because of *Cryptosporidium* contamination.

United States Study finds that more than 30 percent of the U.S. population harbors *Helicobacter pylori*, a bacterium causing stomach ulcers and possibly gastric cancer; MIT researchers uncover bacteria in groundwater.

One of the most important ways to keep your family safe is to pay attention to the reports of food poisoning outbreaks. Keeping up to date with food safety issues gives consumers power.

Keep reading up on the best ways to handle and prepare food; read newspapers, magazines, brochures, and pamphlets on "safe food" topics. When you buy a new refrigerator or stove, carefully read the operating instructions. Many companies are packing the most up-to-date information about how to prevent food poisoning with their appliances. Make sure you know all about your local, state, and federal rules governing safe food in your stores, your restaurants, and all other types of food establishments in your area. Give a call to your local health department if you're not sure. Pay attention whenever the media announce an outbreak of food poisoning or a recall of a food product.

If you suspect food poisoning of any kind, call your doctor immediately!

1

What Is Food Poisoning?

Sue and David Miller woke up within fifteen minutes of each other in the middle of the night, doubled over with stomach pain, vomiting, and diarrhea. All that night and well into the next day, the two suffered with their symptoms.

"It's just a stomach virus," Sue's mother assured her. "It must be going around." But Sue's mother was wrong. The Millers had contracted a severe case of food poisoning after eating commercially prepared meatballs made with raw eggs that were contaminated with *Salmonella* bacteria.

The Millers were fortunate: their toddler had not eaten any of the meatballs, and both of them had been in perfect health before the attack. After feeling miserable for a day and a half, they recovered. For the very young, the very old, and those with weakened immune systems, a bout with salmonellosis can be much more serious.

The important thing to remember is that food

poisoning is not something that occurs only in unclean restaurants or third-world countries. Every day across this country, people prepare, cook, or store food incorrectly, leaving themselves and their families vulnerable to food poisoning.

Food poisoning and food-borne infections are caused by eating food contaminated by toxic substances or bacteria that produce toxins. Usually, a person has to eat food contaminated with certain bacteria, viruses, or parasites before falling ill.

HOW COMMON IS IT?

Food poisoning is one of the most common causes of acute illness. But like the Millers, you may never realize you've been poisoned. Tainted food often tastes and looks perfectly normal, and if you do get sick, you probably assume it's just something that's "going around." Even if you go to the doctor, you probably won't be given the tests that would confirm the cause of your symptoms, and most likely the illness won't ever be reported to public health authorities.

Most food items that carry disease are raw or undercooked foods of animal origin, such as meat, poultry, milk, cheese, eggs, fish, and shellfish. Some four hundred to five hundred food-borne disease outbreaks are reported each year. But not all diseases are likely to be reported, and many cases are sporadic.

Consequently, there is a wide disparity among estimates of the number of food-borne illnesses, ranging from a low of 6 million to a high of 81 million cases yearly, with 9,100 annual deaths, according to the Centers for Disease Control and Prevention (CDC).

At least one-third of the cases have been traced to poultry and meat, but produce (especially imported fruits and vegetables), seafood, and water are other often-contaminated sources. Many types of food-borne infection can also be transmitted directly from person to person if food handlers don't practice good hygiene.

According to the Food and Drug Administration (FDA), just about everyone experiences a food-borne illness at least once a year, whether we realize it or not. Some food-borne diseases, such as botulism and trichinosis, are becoming less common, whereas others, such as salmonellosis, shellfish poisoning, and infection with toxic varieties of *E. coli*, are becoming alarmingly common.

A GROWING PROBLEM

Sometimes it seems that not a week goes by without some scary new report of a food-borne illness that has sickened groups of people somewhere in the United States. It seems as if there are more and more reports of these outbreaks.

In part, this is due to increased reporting. But it's also because Americans now import 30 billion tons of food a year, including fruit, vegetables, seafood, and canned goods, and often we import them from developing countries where food hygiene and basic sanitation are poor. Moreover, the centralization of the food industry means that a single contaminated product may appear in different foods and different forms, potentially infecting a great number of people. If that's not bad enough, new and emerging food-borne pathogens are constantly being identified; these cause diseases that weren't recognized fifty years ago.

Unfortunately, this growing threat to the nation's health comes at a time when microbes around the world are mutating, becoming resistant to modern antibiotics used to combat them. Even now, some strains of enterococcus bacteria have become resistant to the superdrug vancomycin, the antibiotic of last resort.

Your best chance of avoiding illness is to make sure you follow good hygienic rules in buying, handling, and preparing food. But some studies show that too many of us are doing things all wrong: 50 percent of the public admit they eat raw or undercooked eggs; 23 percent eat undercooked hamburger; 17 percent eat raw clams and oysters; and 26 percent don't wash cutting boards after using them for raw meat and poultry.

HIGH-RISK PATIENTS

Many people get food poisoning and barely notice the symptoms, because their healthy immune systems can fight off the infection. For some patients, however, food poisoning is far more serious. Pregnant women are in this high-risk group, especially when it comes to infection with certain bacteria, such as *Listeria*, that target the fetus and can maim or kill an unborn child. The very young and the very old are also at high risk for complications from food-borne illness. Severe diarrhea or vomiting can lead to dehydration, which is a serious health emergency in infants. Infants also can't withstand very high fevers, which may accompany some types of food poisoning. Finally, the physical stress of vomiting and diarrhea can injure sensitive tissues in seniors and babies alike.

People with underlying chronic illnesses such as leukemia, diabetes, or liver disease are at higher risk because their bodies have trouble fighting off infection. People with AIDS are especially vulnerable. What might be a very mild infection in a healthy individual quickly becomes overwhelming for those who can't fight off the attack. In these patients, food poisoning can lead to months of debilitating illness; in the worst cases, it can be quickly fatal.

People who take steroids to treat chronic illnesses, such as asthma, or receive chemotherapy for cancer or organ transplants are at higher risk for food poisoning complications because the drugs weaken their immune systems.

SYMPTOMS OF FOOD POISONING

If you've ever eaten a big meal of chicken or seafood and then gotten sick with diarrhea or vomiting, you've probably assumed it's "just a touch of stomach flu" and let it go at that. Most times, you get better on your own, and you don't think any more about it.

However, keep in mind that *there is no such thing as stomach flu*. Any illness that appears suddenly and within forty-eight hours of eating a high-risk food (e.g.,

Symptoms of Food Poisoning

If you have:	It could be:
Ulcer pain, abdominal pain, fever, nausea/vomiting, diarrhea one week after eating	Anisakiasis
Gastroenteritis, diarrhea, nausea/vomiting 1–6 hours after eating	*Bacillus cereus* infection
Slurred speech, double vision, muscle paralysis 4–36 hours after eating	Botulism
Cramps, fever, diarrhea, nausea/vomiting 1–5 days after eating and lasting up to 10 days	Campylobacteriosis
Nausea, vomiting/diarrhea within 6–12 hours after eating, followed by low blood pressure and heart rate; severe itching, temperature reversal, numbness/tingling of extremities (may last months)	Ciguatera poisoning
Watery diarrhea, nausea/vomiting within hours or up to 1 week after eating; severe cases include bloody diarrhea; infection includes bloody diarrhea and kidney failure	*E. coli* infection
Explosive diarrhea; foul-smelling, greasy feces; stomach pain; gas; appetite loss; nausea/vomiting; incubation period 1–2 weeks	Giardiasis

If you have:	It could be:
Fever, headache, diarrhea, meningitis, conjunctivitis, miscarriage within days to weeks after eating	Listeriosis
Burning mouth/extremities, nausea/vomiting, diarrhea within hours after eating	Neurotoxic shellfish poisoning
Burning mouth/extremities, nausea/vomiting, diarrhea, muscle weakness, paralysis, breathing problems within minutes after eating	Paralytic shellfish poisoning
Diarrhea, rumbling bowels, fever, vomiting, cramps 6–72 hours after eating	Salmonellosis
Itching, flushing, cramps, diarrhea, nausea/vomiting, burning throat; severe infection includes low blood pressure and breathing problems within minutes to hours	Scombroid poisoning
Gastroenteritis, diarrhea, nausea/vomiting 1–7 days after eating	Shigellosis
Explosive diarrhea, cramps, vomiting between 30 minutes and 6 hours after eating	Staphylococcal infection
Diarrhea, nausea/vomiting, fever followed by muscle pain and stiffness 2–3 weeks later	Trichinosis
Gastroenteritis, explosive diarrhea, nausea/vomiting, cramps 8–30 hours after eating (*V. vulnificus* can lead to fatal blood infection)	Vibrio infection

insufficiently cooked eggs, hamburger, chicken, or seafood) and causes stomach pain, vomiting, and diarrhea should be a suspected case of food poisoning. While symptoms vary depending on how badly the food was contaminated, there will often be nausea and vomiting, diarrhea, and stomach pain; in severe cases, there will be shock and collapse.

That's not to say these are the only symptoms of food poisoning. In fact, food poisoning can cause a wide range of symptoms that may not be correctly diagnosed.

While the time between ingestion and onset of symptoms varies according to the cause of poisoning, symptoms usually develop within:

- minutes to several hours for some types of shellfish poisoning
- between one and twelve hours for poisoning by bacterial toxins
- between twelve and forty-eight hours for viral and *Salmonella* infections
- less than thirty minutes in the case of food poisoning by pesticide contamination

Call a doctor if severe vomiting or diarrhea appears suddenly, if the victim collapses, or if you suspect food poisoning and the victim is *a child, an elderly person, or someone with a chronic illness*.

DANGERS FROM FOOD POISONING

Dehydration

The greatest danger from food poisoning is not the toxin itself but the body's natural response to poison—vomiting and diarrhea—which robs the body of vital fluids. This can lead to dehydration and the loss of important elements and compounds called electrolytes (especially sodium and potassium).

It's important to replace these lost electrolytes. You can easily buy replacement fluids designed for this purpose. Drugstores sell electrolytes as clear bottled fluids or in flavored varieties for very young children. Because plain bottled electrolytes have an unpleasant taste, it can be difficult to get children to drink plain varieties. Instead, parents may want to consider buying a packet of flavored electrolyte "popsicles," which can be kept in the freezer and given to the baby or young child when necessary.

If dehydration becomes serious, food poisoning victims may need to be hospitalized and given fluids intravenously.

Complications

While many cases of food poisoning aren't that serious, complications associated with food poisoning are another matter. These complications are much more likely to appear in high-risk individuals than in otherwise healthy adults. They include:

Abortion

Several food-borne infections can have serious consequences for unborn children, including stillbirth and birth defects. Listeriosis is one of the most dangerous food-borne illnesses a pregnant woman can contract, leading to miscarriage or to illness in the newborn baby. Maternal infection with *Toxoplasma gondii* early in the pregnancy can kill the fetus or cause serious brain defects.

Arthritis

Serious problems from a type of arthritis may affect as many as 200,000 Americans each year from food-borne infections caused by *Campylobacter, Salmonella, Shigella,* or *Yersinia*.

Guillain-Barré Syndrome

Campylobacter infection has been linked with the development of this condition—a nerve disease that causes numbness and weakness in arms and legs—and is usually not permanent. However, a small number of patients are permanently disabled, and a few die.

Hemolytic Uremia Syndrome (HUS)

In certain people (usually the very young or old), infection with toxic strains of *E. coli* bacteria may lead to hemolytic uremia syndrome (HUS), a life-threatening complication that destroys red blood cells and causes bloody diarrhea and kidney failure. It was this type of complication to *E. coli* food poisoning from improperly cooked hamburgers that killed several young children in 1993. Implicated in between 2 and 15 percent of infections, *E. coli* bacteria produce a toxin that travels through the bloodstream destroying every major organ it comes to, one by one: kidneys, lungs, pancreas, heart, and brain. In the United States, the toxin-induced condition was once considered rare. Today, HUS is the leading cause of kidney failure in American children, and cases are rising in this country by 3 percent a year. Only in Canada are HUS rates higher.

There is no cure; all doctors can do is wait, moving from one medical emergency to another as the deadly toxin travels from organ to organ. The death rate from HUS is between 3 and 5 percent.

Those who survive HUS struggle with lifelong problems; most are never the same. One-third of the survivors have abnormal kidney function years later and a few need long-term dialysis. Another 8 percent suffer with other permanent complications, such as high blood pressure, diabetes, seizures, blindness, paralysis, or severe brain damage. Others don't live past adolescence, when they outgrow their damaged kidneys. No one can predict what health problems these young survivors may encounter in twenty or thirty years.

Memory Problems

Amnesic shellfish poisoning can lead to confusion, memory loss, disorientation, seizure, and coma within forty-eight hours of eating tainted shellfish (especially mussels). This complication is especially serious with older patients and may appear to resemble Alzheimer's disease. All known fatalities have occurred in elderly patients.

Thrombotic Thrombocytopenic Purpura (TTP)

E. coli bacterial infection in adults may lead to this extremely serious bleeding disorder in which blood stops clotting, small red spots and large bruises appear all over the body, and blood oozes through the mouth. The outlook is not promising for adults who develop thrombotic thrombocytopenic purpura.

TREATMENT

In most cases of food poisoning, symptoms should be treated much like a bout of flu; in particular, liquids (water, tea, bouillon, and ginger ale) should be drunk to replace fluid loss.

Mild cases may be treated at home, with a soft diet, including some salt and sugar. Many cases of food poisoning in healthy adults are not serious (except for botulism, and some types of *E. coli* and shellfish poisoning), and recovery usually takes place within three days.

If food poisoning is suspected, save samples of any food left from recent meals for testing, if possible.

WHEN TO CALL A DOCTOR

You should call a doctor if severe vomiting or diarrhea appears suddenly, if the victim collapses, or if the person experiences numbness and breathing problems.

If you have any suspicion of food poisoning and the victim is a child, an elderly person, or someone with a chronic illness or an impaired immune system, call a doctor right away. Food poisoning in these high-risk people can be serious or even fatal.

HOW TO REPORT SUSPECTED FOOD POISONING

If you think you are ill, first go to a doctor. Then you can think about reporting the illness. According to the U.S. Department of Agriculture's Food Safety and Inspection Service (FSIS), consumers should report possible food poisoning in three situations:

- if the food was eaten at a large gathering
- if the food was from a restaurant, deli, sidewalk vendor, or other kitchen that serves more than a few people
- if the food is a commercial product (such as canned goods or frozen food), since contaminants may have affected an entire batch

Where to Get Help
How do you know whom to call if you have a problem with food or water? The government agency you call depends on the type of problem and the type of food.

Meat, Poultry, or Egg Products:
If you found a strip of metal in a hot dog or a plastic washer in a can of pork and beans, you should call the USDA Meat and Poultry Hotline at 800-535-4555.

Alternatively, you can complain to the store or the product's manufacturer.

Seafood:

The FDA Seafood Safety Hotline number is 800-332-4010.

Nonmeat Food Products:

If you have a complaint about a food product that doesn't contain meat, poultry, or seafood (such as a box of cereal), you should call or write to the U.S. Food and Drug Administration. To find an FDA office in your area, you can check your local phone directory under "U.S. Government, Health and Human Services."

Restaurant Food Problems:

If you think you got sick after eating at a certain restaurant, you should call the health department in your city, county, or state.

Have This Information Ready

When you make a report, officials need to know:

- your name, address, and telephone number
- a detailed explanation of the problem
- when and where the food was eaten
- who ate it
- name and address of the place where the food was obtained

If you want the USDA to investigate a problem about meat, poultry, or egg products, you must have:

- the original package or container
- the foreign object you found (such as a metal piece in a hot dog)
- any uneaten portion of the food (refrigerate or freeze it)

When you call a hotline, be prepared to give this additional information:

- brand name, product name, and manufacturer of the product
- size and package type
- can or package codes (not UPC bar codes) and dates
- establishment number (EST), usually found in the circle or shield near the "USDA passed and inspected" phrase
- name and location of store, and date the item was purchased
- if the tainted food is meat or poultry, the plant where the food was made or packaged (look for the USDA inspection stamp on the wrapper)

2

Buying, Storing,
and Cooking Safely

The first step in protecting your family against food-borne illness is to make sure that the food you buy is the cleanest and healthiest you can find. The government is beginning to crack down on unsafe practices, but there are still plenty of situations where food handling safety can break down. Keep your eyes open and pay attention to the way fresh food is handled, packaged, and presented.

AT THE STORE

As you shop, head for the nonperishables first. Put refrigerated or frozen items in the cart right before you head for the checkout counter. It's important to always check the "sell by" date in the store; obviously, you won't buy anything that has passed this date.

When ordering food at the dairy counter, be sure the clerk observes sanitary practices. If the clerk is handling raw meat or cheese, he or she should be wearing plastic gloves. Don't buy cooked items that have touched raw items in the display case.

If you've ever noticed how raw meat or poultry can drip juices from the package, you'll know you need to protect your other food from this potentially dangerous cross-contamination. Before putting packages of raw meat or poultry in your cart, slip them into plastic bags that you bring along for this purpose.

Don't let the bagger throw your leaking package of chicken breasts on top of the lettuce; make sure any raw food goes into separate bags, away from cooked food and produce. It's a good idea to put all the frozen foods and/or perishable items in the same bags. They'll stay colder—and safer—longer.

During warm weather, when loading your grocery bags, put the perishable items in the air-conditioned car—not the hot trunk. If your grocery store is more than an hour from home, bring along a cooler with ice to store your perishables for the trip home.

Is Your Grocery Safe?

Look for these signs of potential problems when buying meat or poultry:

- frozen meat: white or bleached color (indicates spoilage)
- lamb: brown color
- pork: darkened lean meat and discolored or rancid rind
- poultry: soft, flabby flesh, purplish or greenish color,

abnormal odor, stickiness under wings and joints, darkened wing tips
• thermometer in meat case above 45°F

Be sure to examine the packaging as well.

Packaged Foods

• The package should not be torn, damaged, or opened, or contain spoiled or moldy food.
• Check for: common product name, company/brand name, address of producer or distributor, list of ingredients in descending order of amount present, net weight or volume.

Canned Foods

• Can should have no rust or corrosion.
• Don't buy dented cans, especially if dent affects seal.
• Don't buy leaking, bulging, or swollen cans.

What Do Those Dates Mean?

As you shop, you'll notice a variety of dates on the packages of food. A "sell by" date tells the store how long it can display the product for sale. You should buy the product before the expiration date.

A "best if used by" date is listed as a recommendation for best flavor or quality. It is not a purchase or "safety" date.

A "use by" date is the last date for use of the product while it's at peak quality. This date is a recommendation and has been set by the manufacturer.

Except for the "use by" date, dates that you find on a package don't refer to home storage or indicate how soon you should use the product after you buy it. Even if the date expires during home storage, most products should be safe, wholesome, and of good quality if you've handled them properly. Of course, if the food smells funny or looks odd, it could have acquired some type of "spoilage" bacteria. When in doubt, throw it out.

Keep in mind, however, if you don't store or handle food correctly, bacteria can grow and cause illness even before any "use by" date has passed. If you tote a package of hot dogs to a picnic and leave it in the hot sun, the hot dogs won't be safe to use no matter what date is on the package.

STORE IT!

When you get home, unload the perishables first, and put them in the refrigerator or freezer immediately. If you're going to store meat and poultry in the refrigerator, it's best to leave them in the original packaging (assuming it's clean and not torn). This way, you can keep from contaminating them. Follow any handling recommendations listed on the product, and keep meat and poultry in their packaging until just before you use them.

Never store any food directly under a sink or in cabinets that have water, drain, or heating pipes passing through; food stored here can attract insects and rodents through openings that are hard to seal. Always keep food off the floor and away from cleaning supplies.

Dry Canned Goods

All staples should be kept dry, and stored either in their own packages or in dry, airtight containers. Any moisture that gets into the food (even high humidity) can spoil it. If you notice mold or mildew in the package, the food is spoiled and should be thrown out.

You can keep canned foods stored for a long time at room temperature, but you should still check for expiration dates.

If your cans ever freeze by accident (say, you left them in your car overnight in the middle of winter), you may run into safety problems. Throw it out without tasting it.

If seams have rusted or burst, you'll need to throw the cans out right away. You should also throw out cans that have frozen and then thawed at temperatures above 40°F.

Refrigeration

Temperature in the refrigerator must be 40°F or below. But according to many surveys, lots of folks keep their refrigerators above 50°F. Measure your appliance's cooling ability with a thermometer and adjust the temperature if necessary.

Refrigeration is important to keep your food safe to eat: while cooling doesn't kill bacteria, it stops them from multiplying—and the fewer there are, the less likely you are to get sick.

Allow air to circulate around refrigerated items. To

keep bacteria that's in the air out of the food, always wrap food stored in the refrigerator.

Freezer Facts

If you're freezing meat or poultry in its original package for longer than two months, you should over-wrap the package with airtight heavy-duty foil, plastic wrap, or freezer paper—or place the package inside a plastic bag.

Meat or poultry that has been defrosted in the refrigerator may be refrozen before or after cooking. If you thawed it by another method, you need to cook it before refreezing.

Follow these safe-freezing tips:

- Keep temperature 0°F or below in the freezer.
- Don't stack foods—the cold air needs to reach the center to chill foods fast.
- Freeze poultry and ground meat that won't be used in one or two days; freeze other meat if it won't be used within four to five days.
- If you're going to store meat or poultry longer than two or three months in the freezer, overwrap store packaging with clean plastic wrap or aluminum foil for added protection from freezer burn.

RULE #1: WASH YOUR HANDS!

The single most important thing you can do to keep your food safe is to wash your hands before touching,

Use an Appliance Thermometer

Appliance thermometers are a good way to measure the coldness of your refrigerator and freezer. Refrigerators should maintain a temperature no higher than 40°F, and the freezer should be at 0°F or below.

An appliance device can be kept in the refrigerator or freezer to monitor the temperature—especially important during a power outage.

Cold Storage Guidelines

FOOD	REFRIGERATOR	FREEZER
DAIRY		
Milk	5 days	Don't freeze
Eggs		
fresh (in shell)	3 weeks	Don't freeze
raw yolks, whites	2–4 days	1 year
hard-boiled		
(in shell)	1 week	Don't freeze
liquid pasteurized	3 days	Don't freeze
Mayonnaise	2 months	
(commercial)	(after opening)	Don't freeze
POULTRY		
	Fresh	
Chicken/turkey		
raw	1–2 days	9 months
cooked	3–4 days	4–6 months
giblets	1–2 days	3–4 months
	Cooked Leftover	
Fried/plain chicken	3–4 days	4 months
Pieces covered with		
broth or gravy	1–2 days	6 months
Chicken		
nuggets/patties	1–2 days	1–3 months
CURED PORK PRODUCTS		
Bacon	7 days	1 month
Ham		
fully cooked,		
whole	7 days	1–2 months
fully cooked, half	3–5 days	1–2 months

FOOD	REFRIGERATOR	FREEZER
fully cooked, slice	3–4 days	1–2 months
canned (if label	6–9 months	
says	(unopened)	Don't freeze
"refrigerate")	3–5 days (opened)	1–2 months
Hot dogs		
opened package	1 week	1–2 months
unopened package	2 weeks	1–2 months
LUNCH MEATS		
opened package	3–5 days	1–2 months
unopened package	2 weeks	1–2 months
MEAT (Fresh beef, veal, lamb, pork)		
Chops	3–5 days	4–6 months
Gravy/meat broth	1–2 days	2–3 months
Ground meat	1–2 days	3–4 months
Leftovers (cooked)	3–4 days	2–3 months
Roasts	3–5 days	4–12 months
Steak	3–5 days	6–12 months
Variety meats (tongue, kidneys, liver, heart)	1–2 days	3–4 months
SEAFOOD		
Lean fish, raw	1–2 days	6–8 months
Fatty fish, raw	1–2 days	4 months
Shrimp, raw	1–2 days	9 months
Cooked seafood	3 days	2 months
SOUPS/STEWS	3–4 days	2–3 months
TV DINNERS		3–4 months

Guidelines provided by the USDA and the Food Marketing Institute.

preparing, and eating it, and when cleaning up after it. This simple practice is the single most economical way to prevent contamination. It's simple, it's fast—but you'd be surprised how many people don't do it.

In fact, one recent research team, who stationed themselves in hospital bathrooms and restaurant rest rooms, discovered that not even those people you're counting on to wash their hands do so. Doctors, nurses, food handlers, and servers—many of these folks who should know better—did not wash their hands. Health care workers didn't wash their hands between seeing patients, and food service workers didn't wash their hands after using the toilet.

And yet washing hands has been found to drastically reduce the bacterial and viral counts on your skin. You should wash your hands with soap and water for at least 20 seconds before beginning food preparation; after handling raw meat, poultry, eggs, or seafood; after touching animals; after using the bathroom; after changing diapers; and after blowing your nose.

A good scrub with plain old soap and water will kill about 96 percent of all the bad viruses and bacteria on your skin. You may be surprised to learn that there's a trick to proper handwashing: You should rub your hands briskly for 30 seconds (or the time it takes to sing "Yankee Doodle") in moderately warm water. The rubbing is more important than the type of soap you use (mild soap is fine).

If you wear rings or fake nails and your hands have touched raw chicken parts or hamburger, then you must be sure to scrub the areas around your rings and nails. Soap alone doesn't do a good job of getting under the nail where the microbes are hiding; use a nail file or toothpick to clean under the nails every day. Or better yet, take off your rings and other jewelry before touching raw meat and fish. It makes cleaning up lots easier.

Liquid soap is no better than bar soap, although it may be less messy. But rinsing and drying are very important. Drying is important because the friction of the towel (especially if it's a paper towel) helps remove bacteria and viruses.

WASH YOUR UTENSILS

Wash your cutting board and utensils with hot soapy water before touching food with them. Keep your can opener and blender free from food and particles. Don't season wooden salad bowls with oil; it can become rancid.

Remember that if you wash your dishes by hand, you need to do them all within two hours of putting them in the dishwater. Letting dirty dishes sit in water for a long time creates a bacterial soup, so the contaminants multiply. It's also best to air-dry them.

CLEAN KITCHEN SURFACES

As soon as you finish any stage of cooking, wash your hands and the counters, equipment, utensils, and cutting boards with soap and water.

Food is vulnerable to contamination during storage, preparation, cooking, and serving. Bleach and commercial kitchen cleaning agents are the best sanitizers, provided they are diluted strictly according to product directions; they're the most effective at killing bacteria. Hot-water-and-soap does a good job, but may not kill all strains of bacteria; water alone can get rid of dirt, but not bacteria.

Sanitize Your Surfaces

At least once a week, sanitize your sink, counters, utensils, and cutting boards with a chlorine solution of 2 teaspoonfuls of bleach in 1 quart of water. Let the solution stand before rinsing off. (Always follow the label when using bleach.)

The kitchen sink drain, disposal, and connecting pipe are often overlooked, but food particles get trapped in the drain and pipe, and create an ideal place for bacterial growth. You should sanitize these parts periodically by pouring in a solution of 2 teaspoonfuls of chlorine bleach to 1 quart of water.

Note: Baking soda, lemon juice, and vinegar are popular home remedies for "killing germs" on kitchen surfaces. However, research has shown that they aren't as effective as you may think; they may not leave surfaces germ free.

Sponges/Dishcloths

This may horrify you, but you'll find more fecal bacteria on your kitchen sponge than you will on the rim of your toilet. Time after time, studies of bacteria in the home reveal that the dirtiest, germiest place in your house is the kitchen—and sponges and dishcloths are the worst offenders.

On dry surfaces, bacteria survive for no more than a few hours (although that's long enough to infect food or your hands). But continually moist surfaces, such as cellulose sponges, provide the perfect spot to grow bacteria. Not only is there a good surface to cling to on a sponge, but tiny bits of food supply all the nutrients a bacterium could want. If a sponge stays moist, the bacterial count doesn't decrease for weeks at a time. If bacteria aren't quickly washed away, they can produce an organic glue that cements the cells to the surface, allowing them to survive sprays of water, light rubbing, or even a weak detergent solution.

If you're going to use a sponge or dishcloth to clean your counters, you need to have several: one for the dishes, one to wipe up at the sink, and one for cleaning other kitchen surfaces. Studies have clearly shown that even though you're plunging that cloth into sudsy water, bacteria can thrive. Sponges and cloths should never sit in water, which encourages bacterial growth.

You may want to try a "self-disinfecting" sponge that may grow significantly fewer disease-causing bacteria than an untreated one (ordinary sponges have 450 times more germs than antibacterial sponges). However, it's not clear just exactly how effective antibacterial sponges are, or whether they offer significant extra protection.

Discard sponges for wiping dishes or countertops after one week, or run them through the dishwasher. If you don't have a dishwasher, you can sanitize your sponges by putting them (moist!) into a microwave for one minute. (Don't heat longer than this, or they may burn.)

Alternatively, buy a set of dishcloths and use a clean one each day; put the dirty ones in the wash and run through a hot wash cycle and hot-dry. Or you can dunk the sponge or cloth into a dilute bleach solution. Or use disposable paper towels to clean kitchen surfaces (discard after each use).

Household Cleansers

Cleansers containing chlorine, ammonia, and other corrosive substances are—when used as directed—the best tools against harmful bacteria, viruses, and fungi on your kitchen counters and sinks. While a bucket of water with a cup of bleach added works just as well, it's not as convenient as a spray bottle.

Since no cleanser will be able to disinfect a surface that's covered with dirt, scrub first and then spray with a cleanser. Let the solution stand for as long as the product label advises. (Most won't kill germs on contact; it takes a few minutes. Be patient!)

Remember, when using these products you'll want to wear rubber gloves and ventilate the room. If you have any sort of respiratory condition, including asthma, strong cleansers may trigger breathing problems.

Antimicrobial Products

More than 180 new antibacterial products burst onto the market in 1997—almost five times the number introduced in 1993, according to the Marketing Intelligence Service, a New York State new-product research firm. These products included everything from microbe-shielded scrubbing pads to bacteria-fighting hand lotion, cutting boards, cat-box litter, and bathtub toys.

However, many experts believe that unless you live in a hospital or lab, antimicrobial products aren't that much more effective at removing extra bacteria than plain old soap and water.

Experts also fear that use of these products may end up making germs even more resistant to antibiotics than they already are. Overusing antimicrobials could kill off weaker organisms sensitive to antibiotics, leaving only superbugs behind that are increasingly hard to fight.

CUTTING BOARD SAFETY

While most people believe plastic cutting boards are safer than wooden ones, recent research found that unwashed plastic cutting boards could harbor bacterial growth overnight, whereas wooden cutting boards did not. Whether you use a wooden or plastic board, experts at the University of Wisconsin Food Research Institute urge you to follow these safety tips:

- Wash plastic or wooden boards in hot, soapy water; run plastic boards through the dishwasher. Research shows it's possible to scrub germs from both plastic and wooden boards, except for boards with deeply scarred surfaces.

- Use separate cutting boards regardless of surface for raw meat, seafood, vegetables, and other foods.
- Wash cutting surfaces thoroughly with soapy water and rinse thoroughly between steps in food preparation.
- Sanitize plastic surfaces from time to time with a solution of 2 teaspoonfuls of chlorine bleach to one quart of water. Let the solution sit on the surface for a few minutes, and then rinse with clean water; pat dry.
- To sanitize your wooden board, wet it first and then zap it in your microwave for 10 minutes on high heat; all microbes will be killed (don't microwave plastic boards; their surfaces won't get hot enough).
- When surfaces get deeply pitted or grooved, throw the board out and buy a new one.

TIPS FOR SAFE COOKING

Even if you've bought the best food, stored it correctly, and kept all your kitchen surfaces sparkling and germ free, bacteria can still enter the picture if you let down your guard while you cook. This is an area where lots of folks slip up, especially if they've gotten into the habit of doing things the way their grandparents used to do. Grandma used to reheat the turkey with the stuffing inside ... Grandpop always stored the eggs on the counter and the butter in the cupboard ... Great-aunt Sue always used to press her own cider from windfall apples in the autumn—and she lived to be one hundred and three!

Our ancestors had to cope with a whole different set

of health problems. Today, one of our biggest health crises is food-borne infections, coupled with the rise of new and stronger microorganisms. Scrupulously observing safe food handling practices is the very best way to safeguard your family's health.

Preparing

Whenever you handle any raw food, you should wash your hands before and afterward with soap and water for 30 seconds. If you have an infection or cut on your hand, wear rubber or plastic gloves. But don't think that those gloves absolve you from washing: you must wash as often as if you had bare hands when handling different types of food. The gloves can pick up bacteria just like your skin can. (When washing gloved hands, though, you don't need to take off the gloves and wash your bare hands too.)

Before you open a can, always wash the top with water.

Defrosting

We all defrost food from time to time, but *how* we defrost it can mean the difference between safety and contamination. Defrosting on a counter at room temperature is just asking for the development of bacteria.

Instead, use the refrigerator for slow, safe thawing. Note that different areas of the refrigerator may have different temperatures, and therefore will thaw food at different rates. Also, thawing food on glass shelves seems to take longer than thawing food on wire shelves.

A faster way to thaw food safely is in a cold-water

bath. Thaw sealed packages in cold water, changing the water every 30 minutes. This ensures that the food is kept cold.

The microwave also can be used for safe thawing, as long as you plan to cook the food as soon as it's been defrosted. (See page 45.)

Meat and poultry that have been defrosted in the refrigerator may be refrozen before or after cooking. If they have been thawed by other methods, you need to cook before refreezing.

Using Marinades

Some recipes call for marinating food several hours or overnight, either to tenderize or to add flavor. Marinades can add a great deal to your meal—just be sure to marinate properly so they don't add bacteria as well.

Never set an open dish of food to marinate on your counter while you vacuum the living room or walk the dog. You should always marinate food in a covered dish in the refrigerator.

If you want to use a bit of the marinade as a sauce later, you can separate a small amount of marinade at the beginning before the raw food touches the liquid. Then, serve that reserved marinade as the sauce. Never serve marinade that the raw food had been sitting in, unless you cook the marinade at a rolling boil for several minutes.

Handling Leftovers

If you were to open the door of your refrigerator right now, would you find any bowls filled with furry green mold, or little tufts of white fuzz growing on the leftovers? The main problem with leftovers is that many people put them away and then forget about them until weeks later, when it's not safe to eat them anymore.

There's certainly nothing wrong with saving and serving leftovers, provided you follow the rules to avoid food poisoning.

When you're getting ready to put your leftovers away after a meal, divide the food into small shallow containers to help it cool quicker. Put the food into the refrigerator or freezer promptly. Never refrigerate one large pot of food, or a whole turkey. Once you've wrapped up the food, date it so you can use it within a safe time (usually between three and five days).

It may be helpful to store leftovers in one area of the refrigerator all the time so everyone in the family is accustomed to looking in that section of the fridge for edibles. This will help keep the food from being overlooked, shoved in the back behind the juice, and eventually forgotten.

When it's time to use your leftovers, reheat them thoroughly. Bring sauces, soup, or gravy to a boil, and heat other leftovers to at least 165°F.

Of course, it goes without saying: Throw out any food that looks bad, smells funny, or is covered with mold (except for hard cheese, which may be eaten after you've carefully trimmed off the mold).

Cook Hot Foods Hot: Use a Thermometer

It's important to always cook food thoroughly, since heat will destroy the harmful bacteria. Freezing food or rinsing it in cold water is not enough to destroy contaminants. (Remember—*never* taste food to determine if it's safe. If in doubt, throw it out.)

The only sure way to tell that your food is cooked properly is to use a thermometer. To be safe, a product must be cooked to an internal temperature high enough so that harmful bacteria are destroyed. Many people think that color is the way to tell if food has finished cooking, but recent research has shown that color and texture aren't reliable measures of safety. For example, ground beef may turn brown before it has reached a temperature high enough to kill bacteria. But a burger cooked to 160°F, no matter what color it is, is safe to eat.

You should put the thermometer into the thickest part of the meat or dish (avoiding fat and bone). Check the food in several spots to make sure a safe temperature has been reached, and that harmful bacteria are destroyed. It's especially important not to partially heat food and then finish cooking it later; half-cooked food may be warm enough to encourage bacterial growth but not hot enough to kill it, and subsequent cooking may not kill all the bacteria.

Types of Cooking Thermometers

There are almost as many different kinds of thermometers as there are kinds of food to put them into:

Liquid-filled thermometers are the oldest type of thermometer used in the kitchen. These are designed to be placed in food before it goes into the oven; as the internal temperature of the food rises, the liquid inside the thermometer expands and rises to indicate the temperature on a scale.

Bimetallic-coil thermometers contain a coil made of two different metals that expand at different rates. The coil is connected to a temperature indicator that expands when heated. This type of device senses temperature all along its 2-inch stem; the dial is an average of the food temperature along the stem. These thermometers are available in instant-read and oven-safe types.

Oven-safe bimetallic-coil is the type of "meat thermometer" most familiar to cooks. It's designed to be inserted before the food goes into the oven, and is usually used for large cuts of meat or for poultry. These devices may take as long as a minute or two to show the temperature accurately, but they are a good means of measuring the temperature of thick or deep foods. They are not a good choice for measuring food less than 3 inches thick because the temperature-sensing coil is between 2 and 2½ inches long.

Instant-read bimetallic coil devices are designed to measure the internal temperature of food quickly, and cannot be left in the oven while the food cooks. It takes between 15 and 20 seconds for the temperature to register accurately. You must wash the probe with hot, soapy water after each insertion to prevent cross-contamination. The problem with this device is that it must be inserted full length (usually 2 or 3 inches). If you are measuring a thin food (such as a hamburger), you should insert the probe sideways with the sensing device in the center of the patty.

Check Your Cooking Thermometer

Wonder whether that thermometer is working? Here's an easy way to check. Put a pan of water to boil on the stove (or place a cup of water in your microwave). Once the water has reached a rolling boil, place the stem of the thermometer into the water. If correct, the thermometer will read 212°F.

If it's not correct, look for a calibration nut under the dial that can be adjusted. Most thermometers have one.

Minimum Internal Temperatures

To keep hot foods safe, follow these guidelines from the U.S. Department of Agriculture:

GROUND MEAT

Hamburger	160°F
Beef, veal, lamb, pork	160°
Chicken, turkey	165°

BEEF, VEAL, LAMB
Roasts and steaks

medium rare	145°
medium	160°
well done	170°

PORK
Chops, roasts, ribs

medium	160°
well done	170°
Ham (not precooked)	160°
Sausage (fresh)	160°

POULTRY

Chicken (whole or pieces)	180°
Duck	180°
Turkey (unstuffed)	180°
whole	180°
breast	170°
dark meat	180°
stuffing (cooked separately)	165°

EGGS

Fried, poached	Yolk is white, firm
Casserole	160°
Sauces/custards	160°

FISH
Should be opaque and flake easily with fork

Thermocouple devices are the very fastest thermometers you can buy; they can show a temperature reading on a digital display within seconds. They have
small tips that can accurately measure the temperature
of very thin foods. Since they can be read so quickly,
thermocouple devices can be inserted at several locations to ensure that the food is completely cooked.
This is the type of thermometer used in retail or food
service kitchens.

Candy/jelly/deep fry thermometers are used to measure
food with temperatures ranging from 100°F to 400°F.

Pop-up timers, popular in turkeys and roasting chickens,
are designed to pop up when the right temperature is
reached. The device is made of a food-approved
nylon with a firing material and stainless-steel spring
inside. They have been produced since 1965 and are
accurate to within 1°F or 2°F, if accurately placed in
the product. Experts suggest that you double-check
the temperature with a conventional thermometer in
several places.

Microwaving

What did we do before the advent of microwaves,
when potatoes took an hour to bake, and melting
chocolate was an agonizing process involving numerous pots, water baths, and tedious stirring?

Microwave cooking has certainly been a boon to
busy families and overworked cooks, but there are
unique aspects to this type of cooking that can con-
tribute to bacterial contamination.

Cold spots can occur because of the irregular way the
microwaves enter the oven and are absorbed by the

food. If the food doesn't cook evenly, bacteria may survive and can cause food-borne illness. By following certain basic techniques, you can make sure that meat and poultry microwave safely.

Fast Defrosting

When defrosting with a microwave, first remove the food from the store wrappings. Foam trays and plastic wrap aren't stable at high temperatures, and melting or warping from hot food may promote the transfer of chemical compounds to the cooked food.

Once you have thawed the food in the microwave, you'll have to cook it immediately, since some areas of frozen food may have begun to cook during the defrosting time. Holding partially cooked food isn't recommended, because any bacteria present won't be destroyed.

Follow Instructions

It's important to follow the manufacturer's instructions. Use microwave-safe containers and covers. Use a turntable to rotate dishes as they cook to allow them to cook more evenly. If you don't have a turntable, rotate dishes by hand once or twice during cooking.

Use the Right Dish

High temperatures may cause components of some microwave food packaging materials (such as paper, adhesives, and so on) to enter the food. For that reason, you should choose only microwave-safe cooking containers. Never use the packaging carton for cooking unless the package says you can. Don't use cold-storage containers such as margarine tubs, whipped-topping bowls, or cheese containers. Don't let plastic wrap or thin plastic storage bags touch food during cooking. *Never* use brown grocery bags or newspapers in the microwave.

Microwave Cooking Tips

When you microwave, remember to cover the dish with vented plastic wrap or a lid to hold in moisture and provide safe, even heating. Covering while cooking also helps destroy bacteria. Oven cooking bags also promote safe, even cooking.

Cook large pieces of meat on medium power for a longer time; this allows the heat to penetrate deeper into the meat without overcooking the outer parts. Stir or rotate food once or twice, and turn large food items upside down so they cook more evenly.

When you precook before broiling or barbecuing (see page 49), the healthiest way is to microwave just before popping the food on the grill. You'll reduce the formation of harmful substances if you precook on "high" for 30 to 90 seconds. Make sure to discard the juice.

Be sure there aren't any cold spots in the food where bacteria can survive. For best results, cover the food, stir, and rotate for even cooking.

Reheating

When heating leftovers or precooked food, make sure the internal temperature reaches at least 165°F. Food should be steaming and hot to the touch. Because of the danger of uneven heating, it's not a good idea to reheat baby food or formula.

Testing Your Utensils

Not sure if your dishes are microwave-safe? Put the empty utensil in the microwave beside 1 cup of water in a glass measure. Microwave on high 1 minute. If the dish is cool, it's safe to use in the microwave; if it's hot or warm, don't use.

Barbecuing

When summer comes along, nothing seems more American than firing up the backyard barbecue grill and throwing on a couple of thick steaks. Many Americans believe that nothing beats the outdoor taste of barbecued food. But there are a few things to keep in mind to make sure that food is as safe as possible.

Defrost Before Grilling

Always defrost meat before grilling. When you try to get a piece of frozen meat cooked all the way through, odds are you'll burn the surface.

Charring: Is It a Cancer Risk?

Most Americans have heard those scary stories about contamination from eating undercooked hamburger, and so dedicated barbecuers sometimes think it's a good idea to go in the opposite direction and burn everything to a charcoal crisp.

But don't overdo it—research shows that cancer-causing materials are produced by the actual cooking

Test Your Microwave Oven

All microwaves are not created equal. Ovens vary in power and operating efficiency. Test yours this way:

- Measure exactly 1 cup of cold water into a glass measuring cup.
- Place cup in the center of microwave oven.
- Heat on "high" for 5 minutes, until water begins to boil.
- If water begins to boil in less than 3½ minutes, consider your oven a "high-power" appliance; if it takes longer, the oven is "low-power."

If your recipe calls for a cooking time of 6 to 8 minutes, the high-power oven will do the job in the shorter time (6 minutes), while the low-power oven will take 8 minutes.

of the food on the grill. When flames sear the surface of the meat, carbon in the food is heated in a way that produces aromatic hydrocarbons on the surface. Even if you don't char the meat, high heat can cause substances in the meat to react, producing a group of chemicals that has been shown to cause cancer in animals. While we don't know if these substances are cancer-causing in humans, we do know that all of us are definitely consuming these suspect chemicals when we eat barbecued meats.

This doesn't mean you have to throw away your grill and never barbecue again. But you might want to take the following precautions to minimize your exposure to these carcinogens.

How to Avoid Charring

Microwave your food so that it's partly cooked immediately before grilling. Precooking means the meat will spend less time on the grill, reducing the exposure to processes that create carcinogens. Precooking also removes some of the juices that contain some of the substances that can turn into harmful chemicals during cooking. Also, fewer juices will mean that there is less chance the moisture will drip onto coals, causing higher flames and more charring.

Make sure the food is well on its way to being cooked before you put it on the grill. (And if you do partially cook food in the microwave or on the stove before barbecuing, do so *immediately* before grilling.)

Always grill poultry with the skin on. While it's healthier to remove the skin before cooking poultry on your stove (since the skin is where the fat is), you should leave the skin on when barbecuing and then remove it before eating. That way, you can discard most of the cancer-causing substances that are on the skin. The meat also will be juicier.

When you cook meat and poultry on a grill, the outside often browns very quickly, but that may not mean the inside is completely cooked. How many times have you bitten into a charcoal-grilled hot dog that's nice and charred on the outside, only to find that the inside is completely cold?

Use a meat thermometer to make sure the food has reached a safe internal temperature.

Never partially grill meat or poultry and finish cooking later. Food should be cooked completely once on the grill in order to destroy the harmful bacteria. If you reheat takeout food or fully cooked meats like hot dogs, grill to 165°F (or steaming hot).

Keep It Hot

Once the food comes off the grill, keep it steaming hot until you serve it. If you have a lot of food to barbecue, you can keep the cooked food hot in a 200°F oven while you finish cooking the rest on the grill. After cooking you should hold the food at an internal temperature of 140°F or above.

Once the food is cooked, never put it back on the same platter it was on when it was raw. Any bacteria in the juices could contaminate the safe cooked food. Remember that in hot weather (above 90°F), food should never sit out for more than an hour.

Smoking Tips

You smoke food by grilling slowly over indirect heat in a closed charcoal cooker, adding flavor to large cuts of meat while keeping them tender. It may take up to eight hours, depending on the size of the meat and how cold it is outside. Here are some tips for safe smoking:

- Use good charcoal to build a hot fire.
- Pile about fifty briquettes in the center; when they are covered in gray ash, push them into two piles; place a pan of water between the piles.
- Use wood chips for more flavor (using dry chips in the beginning creates a fast smoke; wet them later for sustained heat).
- Center the food over the water pan and close the lid; keep vents open.
- Temperature in the smoker should be maintained at 250°F to 300°F for safety.
- Add about nine briquettes every 1 to 2 hours.

Canning Safety

There's nothing more satisfying than putting up rows and rows of nutritious, brightly colored fruits and vegetables that you've grown yourself—as long as you can your produce the right way. In the United States, there are about twenty cases of deadly food-borne botulism poisoning annually because people didn't follow the rules.

Botulism is the most serious type of food poisoning there is; it is caused by the rare and very deadly *Clostridium botulinum*. Two-thirds of those affected die, and the rest face a long recovery period, so it's not something you want to mess around with. The bacteria are found in the air, water, and food as harmless inactive spores, until they're deprived of oxygen (for example, inside a sealed can or jar).

Botulism occurs when sealed foods aren't processed at high enough temperatures to kill those toxic spores. The tightly fitted lids of home-canned food provide the anaerobic environment necessary for the growth of the bacteria that produce botulism toxins. The ideal temperature for the bacteria is between 78°F and 96°F; they also can survive freezing.

Fortunately, botulism—and other bacterial contamination in canned food—is easy to prevent, since spores are killed when food is boiled at 212°F for 1 minute during canning or sterilized by pressure-cooking at 250°F for 30 minutes during canning. Moreover, the spores won't grow if the food is very acidic, sweet, or salty (as with canned fruit juice, jams, jellies, sauerkraut, tomatoes, and heavily salted hams).

Salt, sugar, and vinegar are often used in home canning, because these ingredients interfere with the growth of harmful microbes that cause spoilage and food poisoning. For this reason, *you shouldn't change any recipe for home-canned food*. These ingredients are there for a purpose!

There are two methods of canning food: the boiling-water bath and the pressure canner method. The method you select depends on the type of food you're canning.

Check Your Jars

You can't prevent botulism by cooking canned food after you remove it from the container.

Although botulism spores are invisible, it's possible to tell if food is spoiled by noticing the lids; when the spores grow, they give off gas which makes cans and jars lose their seal. Contaminated jars will eventually burst and cans will swell; throw them out.

Check each home-canned jar before opening: if the can is swollen or the safety button in the center of the canning lid has popped up, throw the food away. Any home-canned food with an unusual color should be thrown away *without tasting or even sniffing*.

Jars and Lids

You should only use jars and lids that have been tempered for heat and cold (the mason jar is the most common type). Do not use mayonnaise jars or other commercial jars, or jars with cracks or chips. The two-piece lid (with lid and screw band) is most commonly used today; you can only use the lid once, but the screw band may be reused. Only buy the quantity of lids you can use in one year, because gaskets in older unused lids may not seal.

Boiling-Water Bath

This method can be used to can high-acid foods like tomatoes. The jars of food are completely covered with boiling water—1 or 2 inches over the tops of the lids—and heated for a specific length of time, depending on the food you're canning. (A reliable recipe book will tell you how long to process each food.) Your canner must have a rack to keep the jars from touching each other and to keep them off the bottom of the pot. If the canner is to be used on an electric stove, it should be no more than 4 inches wider than the element on which it is heated. You should not use a large kettle that fits over two burners, because jars in the middle of the kettle won't get enough heat.

Most high-acid foods can be canned this way because they have enough acid to prevent the growth of botulism toxins. However, although tomatoes are considered high-acid, some varieties have less acid than others. For this reason, you should add lemon juice when you're canning tomatoes this way. Two tablespoons of lemon juice should be added to each quart, 1 tablespoon to each pint.

Pressure Canner

The pressure canner is used to can low-acid food such as beets and corn. With this method, jars of food are heated under pressure to a temperature above boiling.

This temperature is needed to destroy the spores of *Clostridium botulinum*, which grow well in this type of food. Process the jars according to the length of time in the recipe.

You must adjust the temperature if you're processing food at altitudes 1,000 feet above sea level or higher. Canners must be cooled at room temperature until they are completely depressurized. Foods can spoil if the canner is exhausted improperly or if canner is cooled too quickly with water.

You should check your dial gauge for accuracy at your county extension office before using your cooker each year. You need to replace the gauge if it reads high by more than 1 pound at 5, 10, or 15 pounds of pressure.

Jelly Making

It's not hard to make safe jams and jellies, provided you follow a few basic rules to minimize bacterial contamination. The most important rule is that when you make jams and jellies, you've got to use the right ratio of fruit, pectin, acid, and sugar. This is not the time to get creative!

Sugar prevents the growth of germs and you should never alter the amount of sugar in a recipe. This is also why you shouldn't double a recipe. Make two separate batches and play it safe.

Because toxic mold can grow on the surface of the jams and jellies, you shouldn't use paraffin or wax seals on top of your jars. Your grandmother might have done it, but it's just not considered safe anymore. Seal jams and jellies with self-sealing lids—just like the ones you

High-Acid/Low-Acid Foods

High-acid foods	Low-acid foods
apples	asparagus
applesauce	beans (shelled)
apricots	beans (snap)
berries	beets
cherries	carrots
cucumbers	corn
fruit juice	hominy
peaches	mushrooms
pears	okra
pickled beets	peas
plums	potatoes
rhubarb	pumpkin
tomatoes	spinach and greens
tomato juice	squash

use for canning fruits and vegetables—and process in a boiling-water bath.

The jam or jelly should be eaten within a few months, or the jelly will begin to lose flavor and color.

Cooking Safely with a Slow Cooker

When it comes to convenience, it's hard to beat a slow cooker. What could be better than walking into an empty house after work and being greeted by a tantalizing smell from the kitchen? In the summer, it can be a relief to use a small appliance and avoid heating up the kitchen with the oven.

Used correctly, the slow cooker is as safe as any other kitchen appliance. This countertop appliance cooks food at a low heat (usually between 170°F and 280°F), which can help to tenderize less expensive cuts of meat. If you follow these guidelines, you don't need to worry about bacteria, since the direct heat, the lengthy cooking time, and the steam from the tightly covered container work together to help destroy bacteria.

Start off with clean utensils and a clean cooker, and follow all the rules for hygienic food preparation. Always defrost meat or poultry before putting it into a slow cooker. Cut food into chunks to make sure it cooks thoroughly. Don't use the cooker for large pieces of meat like a roast or a whole chicken; the food will cook so slowly that bacteria could survive.

Fill the cooker between half and two-thirds full. Put vegetables in first (at the bottom and sides), because they cook slower than meat. Then add the meat and cover with liquid.

If you can, turn the cooker on "high" for the first hour

of cooking, and then adjust to "low." However, it's safe to have the food cooking on "low" the entire time.

If the power goes out while you're away and the cooker is on, throw away the food even if it looks done. It's not worth taking a chance on food-borne illness. But if you're home when the power goes off, you can finish cooking the food immediately in some other way—either on a gas stove or an outdoor grill. If the power goes off while you're there and the food is already cooked, it is safe to leave the food in the cooker with the power off for up to two hours (keep the lid on).

Don't reheat leftovers in a slow cooker. But you can reheat leftovers on the stove (or in a microwave) to a high temperature and then put the food into a preheated slow cooker to keep hot for serving.

Lunch Box Savvy

If your child totes a lunch box to school, you're going to want to be sure that the food is not only nutritious but safe. When packing lunches, remember to keep cold foods cold and hot foods hot. Use an insulated bag, and include a freezer gel-pack for cold food items.

If you don't have an insulated bag, you can use a brown paper sack or a plastic lunch bag, but these won't maintain cold temperatures as well. If you must use one of these, try double bagging; the bags won't get as soggy and can insulate food better.

Some parents like to freeze a juice box and then use that to insulate the lunch; by noontime, the juice has thawed enough to drink, and it's still icy cold. Freezer gel-packs will last until lunchtime, but not all day. If your child brings back perishable food in the lunch box, you shouldn't recycle it for next day's lunch. Throw it out.

If you're sending a hot food—like chili or soup—to school, use an insulated bottle in an insulated lunch box. First, fill the bottle with boiling water, then let it stand for a few minutes, empty out the water, and pour in the hot food. Remind your child to keep the bottle closed until lunchtime to keep the food hot.

Buffets and Special Events

One of the most popular ways to entertain guests is by serving a buffet meal. But whether that's breakfast, brunch, or dinner, the buffet can be a potential source of food-borne illness, since the food is left out for long periods of time.

When serving food at a buffet, be sure to keep hot food over a heat source, and cold food on ice. Refrigerate platters of food until it's time to heat or serve them.

If you're cooking food ahead of time for your buffet, be sure to cook everything thoroughly to a safe temperature. Divide cooked food into shallow containers and store in the refrigerator until you're ready to serve. This encourages rapid, even cooling that can cut down on bacterial growth.

It's Showtime!

When you're ready to put out the food, reheat hot foods to 165°F and arrange them on several small platters instead of one huge one. Keep the rest of the food hot in the oven, or cold in the refrigerator, until it's time to serve it. Serve meat and poultry on a clean plate with

---

Snack Pack

There are plenty of snacks you can pack that don't require refrigeration. These include:

- fresh fruits and vegetables
- cookies
- crackers
- peanut butter sandwiches
- canned meats
- nonrefrigerated cheeses
- packaged pudding
- single-serving canned fruits and juices

a clean utensil to avoid contaminating the cooked food with raw juices found on platters used during cooking.

Remember to keep hot foods at 140°F to 160°F until serving time, especially those served in chafing dishes or warmers. Food should never be kept between 40°F and 140°F for more than two hours, as this encourages bacterial growth.

If you've got hot foods for the buffet table, serve them in chafing dishes, in crock pots, on warming trays—anything to keep the temperature at 140°F or above. Cold food on the buffet table should be held at 40°F or cooler: put the serving dishes in bowls of ice, for example, to maintain proper temperature. If you can't do that, put the food on small serving trays and replace often.

Replenish Carefully

Once your guests have nibbled everything from one plate, don't simply heap more items back onto that same plate. Many people's hands may have taken food from that dish, which has been sitting at room temperature for some time. Put fresh food out on a fresh plate.

Keep track of how long your food has been sitting on the buffet. Perishable food shouldn't stay at room temperature for more than two hours; discard anything that has been around longer than that. Safe buffet time should be cut to an hour if the food is sitting outdoors at temperatures above 85°F.

Buffet Leftovers

At the end of your party, throw out any food that's been sitting around for more than two hours on the buffet table. Other leftovers can be refrigerated or frozen in shallow containers. Most of these leftovers are safe in the refrigerator for four days. They'll keep indefinitely in the freezer, but they'll taste best if used within two to four months.

Mail-Order Food

Especially around holiday times, the mail is full of glossy catalogs offering all sorts of delectable gourmet foods for sale through the convenience of mail order. Ordering a box of cookies, pretzels, or popcorn is one thing, but what about a box of steaks, a honey-baked ham, or a selection of cheeses through the mail? Will the food arrive in good condition and be safe to eat?

It should, if you buy from reputable firms and follow a few simple rules. First of all, when you place your order, ask the company how the food will be mailed. If you're buying a perishable item, it should be delivered as soon as possible—overnight is best. If you're sending the item to someone else as a gift, make sure the words "keep refrigerated" will appear on the box to alert the recipient. You'll also want to find out if there will be instructions with the box about storage and preparation.

If you're sending the package as a gift, tell the recipient that it's coming, and when, if you have a delivery date. This will ensure that your gift won't sit unclaimed outside the house over a weekend, defrosting and spoiling, because the recipient was away. Never send a perishable item to an office unless you can be sure it will be delivered on a workday and there's refrigerator space to keep it cold.

A Word About Lead

When you're serving a buffet, you may like to get out your best lead crystal and Mexican ceramics. But keep in mind that some of the biggest sources of excess lead in our diet comes from using the wrong kind of dinnerware, according to the FDA. If you want to reduce your exposure, follow these tips:

- Don't put acidic foods (such as orange juice) in ceramic containers.
- Limit the use of antique tableware for food and beverages.
- Don't put food or beverages in ornamental ceramic products labeled "not for food use" or "for decorative purposes only."
- Don't store beverages in lead crystal containers for long periods of time.

When you receive an item marked "keep refrigerated," open immediately and check the temperature. With luck, the food will arrive frozen, or partially frozen with ice crystals still visible and refrigerator-cold to the touch. Put the item in the fridge or freezer right away (even if the product is partially defrosted, it's safe to freeze again, although there may be a slight loss of quality).

If It Arrives Warm . . .

If the food arrives warm instead, notify the company if you think you deserve a refund. Do not eat the food. Remember that it's the shipper's responsibility to deliver perishable food on time, but it's your responsibility to have someone there to get the package.

Want to Mail It Yourself?

If you're feeling brave, you can send a perishable item in the mail yourself. Remember that it's best to freeze the item first, and then add a cold source (like a frozen gel-pack or dry ice). Pack the frozen food and the cold source in a sturdy box (corrugated cardboard or heavy foam is best). If there's any empty space, fill it up with crumpled paper or foam popcorn. You want to eliminate any air space in the box that could make the food thaw faster.

Seal the box and label it "perishable: keep refrigerated." Ship your package for overnight delivery, and arrange with the recipient to have someone at home to accept it.

3

On the Road: Safe Food Practices

There's nothing better than packing up the family for a weekend trip, picnic, or camp-out in the fresh air. Or maybe you're getting ready to travel abroad. Should you believe all those stories you've heard about unsafe food and water?

If you're going on the road, no matter where you're headed, it's important to make sure the food you eat is safe.

ON THE MOVE

Many families have discovered the beauty of packing food for long car treks. It saves lots of time and aggravation at crowded rest stops and "fast-food" restaurants that are anything but. As long as you can make sure perishable food is kept cold enough, with a little forethought your trip can be as safe as eating at home.

Plan Ahead and Pack Smart

A well-stocked cooler is a must for long trips. But don't expect to open your fridge on the day you leave, throw a bunch of jars into a box, and be done with it. It takes some planning to be sure that the food you bring along on your trip is safe to eat.

Of course, some foods are naturals that don't require refrigeration, and they are real kid-pleasers: staples like peanut butter, jelly, bagels, or some types of cheese. But if you want to make other types of sandwiches or pack perishable foods like meat, poultry, eggs, fish, or summer salads, plan to keep them in the cooler throughout the trip.

Cooler Tips

Okay, you'll need a cooler, but which one? Most experts recommend foam chests—they're light, economical, and retain the cold very well. However, they may be more fragile than their heavy-duty cousins. So if you're planning on packing some heavy food, you might want to select a plastic, fiberglass, or steel cooler that can take a lot more wear and tear. All these have excellent cold retention, but once filled the larger models may weight more than forty pounds.

If you're planning a long trip, try packing two coolers: one with food for that day's lunch and snacks, and the other for perishables you will use later, or upon arrival. Don't allow anyone to open this second cooler, so as to maintain the cold temperature longer.

If you're going to be using ice in your cooler, remember that a block of ice keeps longer than individual ice cubes. Fill clean, empty milk cartons with water to prefreeze ice blocks, or use frozen gel-packs. Add frozen juice boxes in a variety of flavors. The frozen boxes help keep the food cold; as they thaw, they'll be nice and cool to drink.

Pack the food right from the refrigerator, with food that needs to be kept coldest on the bottom and ice or frozen gel-packs on top. Pack meat and poultry while they're still frozen; they will gradually thaw during your trip, which means they will last longer as you travel. But be sure to separate fish, meat, or poultry so drippings don't contaminate other food. It's a good idea to wrap these potential drippers and then insert them into reclosable plastic bags.

Keep in mind what foods you'll be needing first, and pack in reverse order of use: pack the foods first that you think you'll use last. Wrap everything separately in plastic, and don't place packages directly on ice that's not drinking-water quality. Pack food in the smallest quantity you think you'll need.

Remember that a filled cooler will maintain its cold temperature longer than one that is only half full. If you've packed all you want and there's still space, fill the rest of the space with more ice, fruit, or that extra bag of pretzels or chips.

Carry the coolers in the passenger section of the car, not in the hot trunk. As soon as the ice starts to melt, add more ice. Remember that bacteria grow very quickly at room temperature; throw out any food that warms above refrigerator temperature (40°F).

Keeping Clean

If you won't have access to soap and water, and you don't want to be stopping every few miles, pack lots of moist towelettes to clean dirty, sticky hands and faces. If you use dishes and utensils on the trip and can't wash them, put them all in large-size plastic bags and wash them with hot soapy water when you reach your destination. Remember that one of the best ways to stop food-borne infections in their tracks is to keep your hands clean.

Beverages

Some families prefer to save money by buying larger resealable containers of juice rather than individual juice boxes or cans. If you'll be carrying beverages in larger containers, bring paper cups for all family members; store ice for drinks in a leakproof, resealable container in the cooler. This keeps the ice clean and away from ice being used simply to keep food cold.

At the Campsite

If you're going camping, following a few simple rules will keep everyone healthy even though you'll be preparing and eating food away from sanitary conditions.

When you unpack the cooler, place it in the shade and keep the lid on. (Don't keep the cooler in the trunk of the car.) Insulate the cooler with a tarp, blanket, or poncho.

Keep hot food hot in an insulated dish or vacuum bottle. Keep your utensils and food covered when they are not in use.

Remember that many types of bacteria and viruses

Safe Snacks for the Road

Some snacks are a better bet than others for long road trips. Try offering these, which are crumbless, easier for little hands to manage, and don't carry the risk of food-borne illness:

- fresh fruit
- dried fruit
- soft cookies
- bagels
- carrots or radishes

are transmitted via the fecal-oral route. Clean hands
are imperative when preparing food, so take along disposable wipes to clean hands before and after food
preparation.

Don't leave your food unrefrigerated longer than two
hours (one hour if temperature is above 90°F).

Drinking Water

That bubbling brook may look appetizing, but it's
hard to tell if the water is safe to drink. Bring along
bottled water for drinking or mixing with food. Always
assume that rivers and streams are not safe to drink
from. If you are camping in a remote area, you can buy
commercial purification tablets or equipment, and
learn how to purify your own drinking water.

Cleaning Up

If you don't have access to clean and safe water at
your campground, and you don't have much bottled
water, use disposable wipes to clean your hands when
working with food. Take as few pots as possible, and
plan to cook lots of one-pot meals. Use aluminum foil
wrap and pans for cooking (remember to bring along
garbage bags to carry these things back to a disposal
site). Figure that you may have to bring a camp stove
(many national parks prohibit campfires).

Burn, don't dump, your leftover food. If you are
going to be using soap to clean your pots, wash them at
the camp, not at the edge of the water. Dump dirty water
on dry ground away from any fresh water supplies.

At the Beach

Everybody gets hungry and thirsty during a day at the beach. With a little forethought, it's possible to keep your family healthy and free from food-borne illness.

In addition to all the cooler tips discussed earlier in this chapter, when going to the beach it's important to remember to pack lots of beverages. The best idea is to pack beverages in a separate cooler, since the lid may well be removed often throughout the day. Pack other perishable foods in another cooler; they'll be safer.

Once you've found the perfect spot to spread your towel, set up a beach umbrella and put the coolers in the shade. You may want to partially bury the coolers in the sand, shading them with towels and umbrella.

Perishables should go right back into the cooler after you've eaten; they should not sit out even during the time you run back into the ocean for a brief swim. Remember that perishable food left out of the cooler for more than two hours (or one hour if it's hotter than 90°F) should be discarded.

When you get home, if there's still ice in the cooler and the food didn't sit out for more than an hour, you can save the leftovers. If the ice or gel-pack has melted (or is only cool), don't use any of the perishable leftovers.

Many beaches offer boardwalk dining, with lots of small food stands. When looking for a place to grab a bite, make sure the stand looks clean and well managed. Make sure hot foods are served hot, and cold foods are cold. Don't eat something that may have been sitting out on display in the sun.

Stay Safe: Restaurant Dining

Research shows that you're far more likely to contract a food-borne illness at home than in a restaurant—but that doesn't mean you can't get sick when you eat out. The recent *E. coli* infections at fast-food restaurants are proof that you can.

Of course, it's possible to get food poisoning at even the most elegant eatery, but odds are, the dirtier the restaurant the dirtier the kitchen and the more likely that bacteria will contaminate the food.

Short of inspecting the kitchen yourself, there are a number of ways to assess how careful the restaurant is about cleanliness. First of all, check out the rest rooms. If the bathrooms are dirty, the mirrors are smudged, and there aren't any paper towels in the container, chances are that the kitchen shows the same lackadaisical approach to cleanliness. You'll want to find soap, paper towels or a hot-air blower (not roller towels), clean washbasins, working flush toilets, and a fairly clean floor.

No matter how clean the rest room looks, remember that there may be a host of germs on the fixtures. When using public rest rooms, always turn the faucets on and off with paper towels. Save a clean paper towel to use to open the door as you leave the rest room. If you dry your hands with a hot-air dryer, be sure to wait until your hands are dry so live bacteria don't remain.

In the restaurant take a look at the servers and other workers. They should look clean, with clean hair and nails, and have no open sores, cuts, or wounds. Tables should be clean, as should silverware, glasses, plates, and everything else you can see.

Menu

If the restaurant appears to be acceptable, you can turn your attention to the menu choices. There are some foods that your gastroenterologist would like you to steer away from because of the high risk of contamination: undercooked hamburger, raw oysters and clams, sushi, and dishes made with raw egg (such as Caesar salad).

If you're a healthy young adult and you simply crave sushi, you can take a chance. If you do get sick, odds are you'll survive unscathed after a day or two of discomfort. But if you are pregnant, have a chronic illness (diabetes, asthma, or liver disease, for example), or an impaired immune system, steer clear of any undercooked or raw food. (If you really love the sushi experience, try "vegetarian" sushi, which doesn't include raw fish.)

The most important rule: If you're served an undercooked burger in a restaurant, send it back.

Leftovers

So you've checked out the restaurant, you've ordered healthy, safe entrees—but now what if you've ordered more than you can eat? Most restaurants are happy to offer you containers to tote home food that you can't finish, since you've already paid for it and they can't use it. (However, at least one big-city Boston restaurant refuses to allow patrons to take their food home, for fear of lawsuits if the customers don't store leftovers properly and get sick!)

If you do take food home, you don't have much time to get it safely into the refrigerator, since it's already been lying around on your plate for quite some time. If you don't think you can have it safely refrigerated within an hour of leaving the restaurant, don't bother with a doggie bag. If you're heading to the theater after dinner, do you really want to worry about a soggy bag of filet mignon?

If you do go right home and get the food in the fridge, remember to eat it within twenty-four hours or throw it out. If you're reheating it, make sure it reaches a temperature of 160°F (185° in the microwave).

Salad Bars

If you've ever approached a salad bar and watched other diners mangle the lettuce and touch food with their bare hands, you'll understand why the government established guidelines for public self-serve food areas.

Meat and poultry products on display must be protected from contamination by a counter, service line, or salad-bar food guards. Unpackaged, raw meat can't be offered for consumer self-service. But use your head: if the food on the salad bar looks lifeless, brown, and shriveled, or if it has a funny smell or taste once you get it back to your table, don't eat it. Either wait until the workers replenish the salad bar with fresh food, or skip it.

INTERNATIONAL TRAVEL

While stomach problems aren't inevitable as soon as you leave the borders of the United States, it is true that

Hand-Washing Hygiene

Soon infrared devices may alert companies whose employees aren't washing their hands correctly. The new Hygiene Guard system is an infrared detection system that alerts the employer whenever workers leave the rest room without washing their hands.

It's being tested at the Tropicana Hotel in Atlantic City and at several medical centers around the country.

contaminated food and water are a problem for travelers, especially in areas of poor sanitation. Fortunately, there are things you can do to protect yourself when traveling abroad.

Water

When you're traveling, remember that even chlorination won't protect you against some enteric viruses and the parasitic organisms that cause giardiasis and amebiasis. In areas where you know sanitation leaves something to be desired, these beverages are the only things safe to drink:

- boiled water
- hot beverages made with water that has been boiled, like coffee or tea
- canned or bottled carbonated beverages
- beer and wine

Don't use ice that may have been made from unsafe water. If you're drinking directly from a can or bottle, wipe it off first so that it's clean and dry, because water on the surface of the container may be unsafe. Don't brush or rinse your teeth with water that may be contaminated.

Treating Water

You can boil water to make it safe and then allow it to cool on its own before drinking (don't add ice to cool it down). If you're at a high altitude, boil vigorously for a few minutes, or use a chemical disinfectant. To improve the taste, you can add a pinch of salt, or you can pour the water from one container to another.

You can chemically disinfect water with either iodine or chlorine (iodine will protect you against more contaminants). Specially designed chemical disinfection products can be bought in sporting goods stores, camping outlets, and pharmacies.

If the water you're treating looks cloudy, strain it through a clean cloth and then use twice the amount of disinfection tablets you ordinarily would. (If the water is very cold, the disinfection won't work as quickly; either warm the water or wait longer for the disinfection to work.)

If you must use tap water and can't disinfect it, then tap water that's very hot to touch is marginally safer—but it still could contain many disease-causing microbes.

Food

When you're traveling abroad (especially in areas with poor sanitation), keep in mind that any raw food you eat could be contaminated. There are a number of foods that are particularly risky, including salads, uncooked vegetables and fruits, unpasteurized milk and milk products, raw meat, and shellfish.

Fruit that you can peel yourself is probably safe, as is food that has been cooked and is still hot. However, note that some fish may not be safe even if it is cooked to a crisp because of toxins in the flesh. This includes fish such as red snapper, grouper, and sea bass, if they are caught on a tropical reef instead of in the open sea.

Highest-risk areas are the West Indies and the tropical Pacific and Indian Oceans.

Traveler's Diarrhea

Diarrhea is the major health problem among travelers who journey to developing countries. If you're going to a high-risk area (Latin America, Africa, the Middle East, or Asia), the risk of getting diarrhea is between 20 and 50 percent.

The diarrhea is caused by consuming water or food that is infected, primarily with *E. coli*, although a host of other microbes have been implicated.

If you want to try to prevent traveler's diarrhea, in addition to monitoring food and drink, you can try taking bismuth subsalicylate (Pepto-Bismol) before you get sick. Take 2 ounces four times a day, or 2 tablets four times daily (but don't take it for more than three weeks). There may be some side effects, including a temporarily blackened tongue, black stools, occasional nausea and constipation, and perhaps ringing in the ears. Ask your doctor before you leave if you can take this drug (some people shouldn't take Pepto-Bismol).

If you're on the pessimistic side—or you just like to be prepared—you might want to ask your doctor for a prescription antibiotic to take along for traveler's diarrhea, just in case. This way, if you do come down with diarrhea, you won't have to worry about finding a doctor in a foreign country when you're feeling lousy. Having an antibiotic available at the first sign of illness can cut the number of days you're feeling ill.

If, despite all your efforts, you get sick anyway, you

may be comforted to know that if you're young and otherwise healthy, your condition is probably not life-threatening. That doesn't mean you won't feel very sick; in addition to diarrhea, you may have nausea, bloating, and malaise that can last from three to seven days.

The risk of infection varies depending on where you eat: a private home is low-risk, but a street vendor is asking for trouble.

While you're sick, avoid dairy products and try to drink plenty of liquids (safe ones!). Children or infants who are sick with diarrhea should be taken to a doctor immediately, since dehydration can be a serious problem in this age group.

Cruising Safely

The pictures of those seagoing buffets look marvelous, but just because a cruise ship is floating in the middle of the ocean doesn't mean it's safe from bacterial contamination. Remember that a ship loads fresh fruits and vegetables in some very risky parts of the world. Because cruise lines have had major disease outbreaks in the past, the CDC has set up a program to monitor cruise ship safety and protect passengers.

Basically, every ship that carries more than thirteen passengers and makes stops abroad must have twice-yearly inspections at U.S. ports, including a review of employee hygiene, general cleanliness, and potential contamination of food, water, and ice. A ship that earns a score of 86 or above has passed; the lower the score, the lower the level of sanitation.

If you're getting ready to take a cruise and you

wonder how sanitary your liner is, you can obtain a copy of the ship's most recent sanitation inspection report by writing to: Chief, Vessel Sanitation Program, National Center for Environmental Health, 1015 North America Way, Suite 107, Miami, FL 33132.

4

Disaster:
Are You Prepared?

Most times, you have some warning that a hurricane or flood is heading your way. While most of us are worried primarily about keeping our family physically safe and protecting our homes at a time like this, in the wake of the disaster we often overlook something equally important: safeguarding our food and water supplies. Or as we struggle to clean up after a flood or hurricane has damaged our house, we may not be sure whether that dented can or damp sack of flour should be saved or thrown away.

PLAN AHEAD

Advance preparation is the key to keeping your food safe in the event of some type of natural disaster. If you know that you live in an area prone to hurricanes, earthquakes, tornadoes, or floods, it pays to keep adequate supplies on hand, because power will likely be disrupted at one time or another.

Before a Power Outage

The most likely problem you'll have to cope with in severe weather is a power outage. Especially in rural areas, with wide open spaces and long expanses of power lines strung between poles, it seems as though every storm knocks out power for a few hours.

If you often lose electricity during storms, you can prepare for the next situation to keep your food as safe as possible. Here's what you can do:

- Stock up on nonperishable things, such as canned food, juice, and "no freeze" dinners in paper cartons.
- Find out ahead of time where you can buy dry and block ice (check the Yellow Pages).
- Buy some gel-packs and keep them frozen, or freeze water in plastic containers.
- Buy a cooler.

Before a Flood

If you live in an area that is prone to flooding, you should be prepared to raise your refrigerator or freezer (put cement blocks under the corners). Canned goods and other food kept in low cabinets or the basement should be moved to higher areas in the home.

Emergency Supplies to Keep on Hand

- enough nonperishable food and water for four to five days
- manual can opener
- battery-powered radio
- extra batteries
- camp stove and fuel (or other emergency cooking equipment)
- flashlights, candles, matches, kerosene lamp
- fire extinguisher
- first-aid kit

WHEN DISASTER STRIKES . . .

If You Lose Power

Everyone who has ever sat through an electrical storm in the dark, wondering about that freezer full of food thawing in the basement, may be happy to learn that a full freezer can stay cold enough for about two days without electricity; a half-full freezer lasts about one day. An unopened refrigerator should keep food safely cold for about six hours, depending on the room temperature.

When your electricity does go off, it's important to keep the freezer and refrigerator closed. You don't need to open the door to check if the food is still cold—it is, at least for the first few hours, if you don't open the door.

Long-Term Power Loss

If you have reason to believe that power won't be coming back on for more than two days, try to find some dry ice for the freezer. If you haven't checked this out beforehand, call the power company. It may have sources of dry ice, or it may provide dry ice to customers at central pickup locations in a disaster situation. (Stay tuned in on your battery-powered radio to find out.)

Follow the handling instructions carefully (remember, dry ice burns). Dry ice is cold: $-216°F$. Wear heavy gloves with no holes, and use tongs. Neither touch the ice with bare skin nor breathe its fumes in an enclosed area. About 25 pounds of dry ice should keep a 10-cubic-foot full freezer cold for up to four days.

While dry ice can also be used in the refrigerator,

block ice is better here. Put the block into the refrigerator's freezer unit, and place all perishable items (meat, poultry, dairy) in there. Group meat and poultry to one side or on a plate so that as they begin to thaw, their juices won't contaminate other food.

Once your food starts to thaw, you'll need to check each item to decide what is safe to keep. Normally, you need to be very careful about meat or poultry, or any food containing milk, sour cream, or soft cheese.

Raw meat and poultry from the freezer can usually be refrozen without too much loss in quality. Prepared food, vegetables, and fruits can normally be refrozen after a power loss, but they may lose some quality. Refrigerated items should be safe as long as the power hasn't been off for more than a few hours. If the power remains out for more than two days, freezer food may have to be thrown out.

After a Flood

If flood waters have entered your house and come in contact with your food, anything they have touched is probably dangerous to eat. Flood waters often carry silt, raw sewage, and chemical waste into homes. They are notorious for bacterial, viral, and toxic contamination, with everthing from cholera to *E. coli*.

When in doubt, throw it out.

Check food and throw out any with slivers of glass or other debris.

You can probably save commercially canned goods if they aren't damaged or dented, and if you sanitize the cans. Here's how:

What's Not Safe in the Refrigerator

Discard if held above 40°F for more than two hours:

bacon
beef (dried)
casseroles
cheese (soft)
cottage cheese
cream
egg dishes
eggs (fresh or hard-boiled)
fish (fresh or leftover)
garlic (chopped, in oil or butter)
gravy
hams, canned (labeled "keep refrigerated")
hot dogs
lunch meat
meat (fresh or leftover)
milk
pasta (cooked)

pasta salads with mayonnaise or vinegar base
pastries (cream-filled)
pies (custard, cheese-filled, or chiffon)
pizza with meat topping
potatoes (baked)
poultry (fresh or leftover)
refrigerator biscuits, rolls, cookie dough
sausage
seafood (fresh or leftover)
soups
sour cream
stews
stuffing
yogurt

What About Frozen Food?

Discard everything if thawed and held above 40°F for more than two hours, except for:

breads, rolls, muffins: refreeze
bread dough (commercial or homemade): refreeze, but quality may be lost
cakes without custard fillings: refreeze
cheese (hard): refreeze
cornmeal: refreeze
flour: refreeze
juices: refreeze, but discard if mold, yeasty smell, or sliminess develops
nuts: refreeze
piecrusts: refreeze

- Mark contents on can lid with indelible ink.
- Remove labels (paper can harbor dangerous bacteria).
- Wash cans in strong detergent solution using a scrub brush.
- Immerse containers for 15 minutes in a solution of 1 teaspoonful of chlorine bleach per quart of room-temperature water.
- Air-dry before opening.

You should also be sure to sanitize all dishes and glassware the same way you sanitize cans. To disinfect metal pans and utensils, boil them in water for 10 minutes. *Discard all wooden spoons, plastic utensils, baby bottle nipples, and pacifiers.*

Discard These Foods

Throw out any of the following foods that have come in contact with floodwater: all meat, poultry, fish, and eggs; fresh produce; jams or jellies sealed with paraffin; home-canned food; commercial glass jars of food or beverages, including sealed jars with corks, pop-tops, peel-off tops, or waxed cardboard seals (such as mayonnaise and salad dressing); all food in cardboard boxes, paper, foil, cellophane, or cloth; spices, seasonings, and extracts; open containers and packages; flour, sugar, grain, coffee, other staples in canisters; cans that are dented, leaking, bulging, or rusted.

Water: Is It Safe?

After a flood, you should probably figure that most of the water is unsafe to drink. Before you turn on that tap for cooking, cleaning, or bathing, wait until local health authorities tell you it's not dangerous. If you absolutely have to use the water from the tap, boil it first for 1 minute (up to 5 minutes if you live at a high altitude).

Cleaning Up After a Flood

It's extremely important to clean and disinfect your kitchen after it's been contaminated with floodwater. Start with warm, soapy water, and scrub the kitchen counters, pantry shelves, refrigerator, stove, and all dishes and glassware. Then follow that with a rinse of chlorine bleach solution (2 teaspoonfuls per quart of water), using a fresh cloth.

After a Fire

If your house has been damaged in a fire, throw out any food that has been near or exposed to the fire, since the heat can cause damage and toxic fumes can contaminate food. Throw out food even if it was in the refrigerator or freezer, since these appliances aren't necessarily airtight; toxic fumes may have reached the food inside. Even canned goods can be spoiled if they were close to heat and flames, because the heat could have activated bacteria inside the cans.

The toxic fumes released during a fire can contaminate all types of food in permeable packaging (that's cardboard, plastic wrap, and so on). If you had any foods sitting on the counters, such as apples or bananas in a bowl, they should be discarded.

5

Beef, Lamb, and Pork

Jared was a laughing blond five-year-old dynamo who loved Power Rangers and fast-food restaurants. Then he almost died from eating a hamburger contaminated with the same deadly bacteria that caused a devastating 1993 outbreak in the Pacific Northwest. His kidneys failed. He needed blood transfusions to combat anemia. Seizures racked his body. Fluid filled his lungs. His veins collapsed. Miraculously, two months in the hospital and $75,000 later, he recovered. Doctors still don't know how.

But he is not the same. He had to learn to walk all over again, and his kidneys and blood must be checked every three months. His parents will never know if his mental abilities have been permanently damaged. He still talks about dying.

Chances are, when you think of food poisoning you think of the notorious "hamburger disease" that sickened and killed youngsters at several fast-food restaurants in the early 1990s. It was that image of a child struck down from eating something so all-American as a burger and fries that changed the way we looked at the problem of food-borne illness and bacterial contamination, and it jolted the U.S. government into the first overhaul of its meat inspection system in a century.

For many parents across the country, it came as a shock to realize that food poisoning was no longer a problem of third-world countries' bad water and poor sanitation. It was everybody's problem.

E. COLI

The "hamburger disease" is caused by a lethal strain of *Escherichia coli*, the bacterium that normally lives harmlessly in the human intestine. The new strain, *E. coli* 0157:H7, is found in cattle feces, and when ingested by humans, it can produce a powerful toxin that causes severe illness.

In the last few years, the Centers for Disease Control and Prevention have received reports of this disease in twenty-three states. CDC experts estimate that this one type of bacteria alone may be responsible for at least twenty thousand illnesses and up to five hundred deaths a year in the United States, and they suggest that the true incidence may be much higher. Because in most cases doctors are not required to report this type of poisoning, there is no way of knowing for sure just how many hundreds of other Americans have died from the same disease.

Many government experts consider the disease to be

an epidemic on the upswing, and they think that what we're seeing is the nation's major emerging infectious disease.

How It Occurs

Bacteria are everywhere in our environment, and any food of animal origin can be contaminated with it. Some bacteria will spoil food, giving it an unpleasant taste or smell, but won't cause illness. Other bacteria can make you very sick. Grinding exposes more of the meat surface to bacteria, which is why hamburger is so often implicated in food-borne illness. This type of food poisoning appears to be increasing, as has the frequency of complications from infection.

Meat becomes contaminated during slaughter. Because of the centralization of the U.S. beef industry, it takes only one infected animal to contaminate huge amounts of hamburger as the ground meat is mixed in one-ton vats. (Alternatively, bacteria on a cow's udders or on milking equipment can find its way into raw milk.)

Since the tainted meat usually looks and smells normal, it's possible to eat it unknowingly. Although the number of organisms needed to cause disease isn't known for sure, it's believed to be very small; scientists estimate that as few as one to ten *E. coli* organisms can kill a child. Several thousand of them can fit on the head of a pin. Once meat has been contaminated, without proper refrigeration the number of bacteria doubles every four hours.

Unfortunately, if another outbreak did occur, there's

a good chance you would never find out about it, since most cases of *E. coli* poisoning are not officially counted by the CDC. Some states do not report individual cases of *E. coli* poisoning. Others don't report at all. In fact, the only reason most people have heard about the poisonings linked to a Jack-in-the-Box restaurant in Seattle, Washington, is that the disease affected so many hundreds of people that word leaked out.

The disease was first recognized as a cause of illness in 1982 during three separate outbreaks of bloody diarrhea that were traced to contaminated hamburger. The strain continued to appear sporadically in different parts of the country until 1993, when four children died and hundreds more became ill after eating *E. coli*–tainted hamburger in a Seattle fast-food restaurant. The Seattle outbreak was followed within months by more outbreaks of food-borne illness caused by *E. coli*; these forced the closing of two other restaurants and sickened sixty more consumers.

A child can become ill from eating a contaminated hamburger at a local fast-food restaurant, but he also could pick up the illness from his mom if she makes hamburgers at home with raw meat, wipes her hands on a dish towel, and then uses the towel to wipe the child's face. Day care workers touching contaminated burgers or the diapers of infected infants can go on to contaminate every toy and surface they touch. Every child in the center who touched the toys could then become infected.

Figures from the Centers for Disease Control suggest this bacterium may cause 20,000 illnesses a year in this country, with 250 to 500 deaths from *E. coli* 0157:H7 alone.

This is not a problem that occurs only within the borders of the United States. In the summer of 1996, a similar epidemic that swept through Japan killed seven people and infected almost nine thousand during a four-month epidemic.

New Hope for Prevention

The horror of these epidemics was not lost on the federal government, which was jolted into an attempt to prevent future occurrences.

The USDA developed a new ten-minute test to determine potentially dangerous *E. coli* bacteria in meat. The test is now available to the wholesale food industry. A test that consumers can use may soon be available.

OTHER TYPES OF MICROBES IN MEAT

Unfortunately, *E. coli* is not the only contamination that you may find in your meat. "Hamburger disease" is only one of an ever-growing array of food poisoning bugs that may contaminate beef and cause food poisoning; these include *Salmonella*, *Campylobacter*, *Listeria*, *Staphylococcus*, and *Clostridium perfringens*.

Most people think that *Salmonella* is found exclusively in eggs and poultry, but in fact it also may be present in other types of meat, causing intestinal upsets that can be severe in certain high-risk people. *Salmonella* is not destroyed by freezing, but it is killed by thorough cooking. *Staphylococcus aureus* can contaminate meat handled by an infected food preparer; most outbreaks are transmitted this way. Sanitary food handling and proper cooking and refrigeration can prevent this illness. *Clostridium perfringens* infection is a mild food-borne illness caused by multiplying toxins; it is commonly found in meat that hasn't been cooked well enough. *Listeria* is a type of bacteria that can contaminate ready-to-eat products such as salami, beef franks, and lunch meat. It is a problem for high-risk people and pregnant women. Be sure to refrigerate these products well and observe the "use by" date on the label.

Mad Cow Disease

A special problem for those who love beef is the concern about bovine spongiform encephalopathy (BSE), known popularly as "mad cow disease," which was identified in British cows in 1986. It seems to be one of a group of diseases that take different forms in different species, including the human form of the disease, Creutzfeldt-Jakob disease (CJD), a type of spongiform encephalopathy that causes severe dementia and is always fatal.

Mad cow disease and CJD seem to be related: both attack and destroy the brain in the same way, leading to the formation of numerous holes in the brain until the tissue resembles a sponge. In cows, mad cow disease causes behavioral changes, weakness, loss of coordination, and death.

BSE is believed to have infected British cows when they ate cattle feed that included sheep offal contaminated with scrapie, the ovine version of BSE. The world's attention was focused on Britain in the 1990s when cases of CJD in Britain nearly doubled from 1990 to 1994, reaching fifty-five cases. Concern heightened when a cluster of twelve more British cases of a variant form of CJD were diagnosed in 1996. By the end of 1997, another eight cases had been reported.

Recent research suggests that the cause of the BSE in the British cattle is the same as that of the new type of CJD in people, and that the British cases were indeed related to contaminated beef. However, no one knows for sure if these cases are an isolated cluster, or the forerunner of an epidemic among those who ate BSE-contaminated beef in England in the 1980s.

There have been a few sporadic cases of CJD in other countries that had infected cattle, but no evidence of higher risk in the United States or Canada. In fact, the USDA maintains that BSE doesn't exist in the United States. In 1989 the USDA banned beef imports from countries where BSE has been reported. The number of CJD cases in the United States has remained stable at one per million since 1979.

The infectious agent of these diseases is believed to be a prion, an unusual infectious agent that is neither bacteria nor virus, and can't be destroyed by normal means, including ionizing radiation or even boiling at temperatures well over 400°F.

Since 1988, the British government has set up much stricter regulations regarding tainted beef, including slaughter of exposed cattle and a ban on using some types of offal (especially the brain) in animal feed. As a result, there has been a major drop in the incidence of BSE in British beef over the last few years.

HORMONES AND ANTIBIOTICS

While contamination with microbes is a primary concern with beef, pork, and other types of meat, many consumers also worry about eating meat that may contain hormones or antibiotics.

Antibiotics are given to prevent or treat diseases in cattle, much as in humans. Although penicillin is not used in beef cattle, tetracycline has been approved (but isn't widely used). Hormones—including estradiol, progesterone, and testosterone (three natural hormones), as well as synthetic hormones—may be used to promote growth.

Farmers must observe a "withdrawal period" between the time antibiotics are given and the time the animal goes to slaughter, and the government randomly samples animals at slaughterhouses to test for residues. But of the millions of cattle, hogs, and sheep slaughtered each year, only a fraction are inspected for residues.

Critics worry that using hormones and antibiotics in animals intended for human consumption may mean medications may still be in the meat after the animal is slaughtered. Long-term risks of meat containing antibiotics are not known. And while meat producers argue that the amount of hormones in meat is very low, it doesn't take very high doses of exogenous hormones to adversely affect human health.

Consumers who wish to avoid antibiotics and hormones in meat may want to consider buying meat from small or organic farms that raise animals without using hormones or antibiotics.

WHAT YOU CAN DO

When it comes to avoiding food poisoning in beef and other types of meat, there is a great deal that you can do to protect yourself, starting with making wise choices at the market.

First of all, make sure that all beef, pork, lamb, and veal you buy has been inspected and graded by the USDA. Choose your meat right before heading to the register to pay. Put raw beef in disposable bags if you can, so it doesn't drip onto any other food. Select packages that aren't torn, and that feel cold. The meat surface exposed to air will be red; interior fresh meat will be dark. Have the checkout clerk put your raw meat, poultry, and fish in a bag separate from the rest of your purchases.

STORING BEEF AND OTHER MEATS

When you get your meat home, be sure to refrigerate or freeze it immediately so as to stop the growth of bacteria. Use it between three and five days after buying if you have not frozen it. Observe the "use by" dates. Cook-before-eating hams have been treated to destroy organisms, but they still must be fully cooked at home within seven days.

Freezing

You can safely freeze beef in its original package, or you can repackage it for storage. However, if you're going to keep the beef in the freezer for a long time, it's a good idea to overwrap the store packaging with plastic wrap, aluminum foil, freezer paper, or plastic bags made for freezing to prevent freezer burn (this appears as grayish-brown spots and is caused by air touching the food surface).

Freezer burn won't hurt you, but the meat won't taste as good. You can cut off freezer-burned sections of meat before or after cooking. For best results, use steaks and roasts within nine to twelve months. Mark the packages so you can keep track.

Freezing pork kills pork tapeworm and roundworm; keep at 5°F for thirty days to kill roundworm cysts, and four days to kill tapeworm cysts. For maximum quality, don't freeze hot dogs any longer than a month or two.

DEFROSTING

Never defrost any meat product on the counter at room temperature. You can safely defrost in the microwave, in the refrigerator, or in a cold-water bath.

Refrigerator Defrosting

If you choose this method, it will take a day to defrost ground beef, stew meat, or steaks. Bone-in meats and whole roasts may take two days (or even longer).

Once the raw beef defrosts, you must cook it within

three to five days. If after this time you decide not to cook it, you can refreeze it without cooking first.

Cold-Water Bath

If you want to defrost your beef in a cold-water bath, don't take off the wrapping. Be sure the package is airtight, or put it in a leakproof bag. Submerge in cold water and change the water every half hour. It may take an hour or less to defrost small packages of beef, but a three- or four-pound roast could take two or three hours.

Microwave Defrosting

If you're going to defrost beef in the microwave, be sure to cook it right afterward, because some of the meat may already have begun to cook. Holding partially cooked food isn't recommended because the bacteria won't be destroyed. Foods defrosted in the microwave or by the cold-water method should be cooked before refreezing, because they may have been held at temperatures above 40°F.

PREPARING

Always wash your hands thoroughly in hot, soapy water before preparing food and then wash everything that touched raw meat. Wash hands, utensils, counters, cutting boards, and sinks afterward with hot, soapy water.

Marinating

You can marinate beef in the refrigerator for up to five days. If you're going to use any of this marinade later on cooked beef, be sure to boil the marinade first. Throw out any unused marinade.

Microwaving

If you're trying to microwave unequal pieces of beef, arrange them in a dish so that the thick parts are toward the outside of the dish and the thin parts are in the center. If you're microwaving a roast, put it into an oven cooking bag or a covered pot. Use a meat thermometer to test for doneness in several places, and to make sure correct internal temperatures have been reached.

It is safe to microwave burgers, but since microwaves may not cook food as evenly as other methods, it's a good idea to cover burgers while they cook to help them heat evenly. Allow patties to stand for 1 or 2 minutes to complete cooking.

COOK IT!

When you cook meat, it's important that you keep the temperature high enough long enough to kill bacteria. The USDA recommends that you:

- Cook burgers and ground beef mixtures (such as meat loaf) to 160°F.
- Cook steaks/roasts (whole-muscle meats) to 145°F

(medium rare), 160°F (medium), or 170°F (well done).

- Cook pork to 160°F (medium) or 170°F (well done).

Roasting

One of the best ways to cook tender meats (such as beef tenderloin or standing rib roast) is to roast them in a moderately low oven at 325°F. The meat is placed on a rack in a shallow, uncovered pan and cooked by indirect dry heat. The low temperature keeps the meat tender and minimizes shrinkage due to moisture evaporation. However, meat should never be roasted at any lower than 325°F or harmful bacteria could multiply.

Insert the thermometer in the roast's midsection, avoiding the bone. If the food is irregularly shaped, check the temperature in several places.

Because beef roasts are muscle meats, any bacteria would most likely be on the surface; for this reason, a beef roast doesn't need to reach 160°F in the center to be safe.

Hamburger

The problem of *E. coli* contamination occurs primarily with hamburger, because, as mentioned earlier, when contaminated beef is ground and mixed with other beef, the bacteria become widely distributed— not just on the surface, but throughout the meat. When you realize that in many slaughterhouses hamburger is mixed in one-ton vats that are then shipped to all parts of the country, it's easy to see how the problems start. The toxin-making bacteria are killed only if the hamburger is cooked to an inside temperature of 155°F, hot enough to eliminate all meat pinkness.

While it's possible to become very, very sick from contaminated meat, the good news is that simply by following safe cooking practices, you should be able to avoid problems.

The most important thing you can do is cook all hamburger until it is well done with no pink color and the juices run clear. Cooking kills all the harmful microbes that typically contaminate meat, so if you are careful at this stage of preparation, you can feel sure you're protecting yourself and your family against food-borne illness.

Use a thermometer to make sure hamburger is cooked to 160°F; insert into the thickest part of the hamburger. Since it's hard to cook thick patties completely, make thin ones and slit the middle to make sure the inside is brown. If you're having trouble inserting a thermometer into a thin patty, pierce the patty sideways.

Once burgers are cooked, never put them back on a plate that held raw patties. Never use cooking utensils you've just used for raw meat with other food, and wash your hands thoroughly after handling raw meat. Never taste or eat raw beef or any other meat as you cook it.

Pork

Because hogs are about 50 percent leaner than their ancestors were twenty-five years ago, today's pork may dry out when it's overcooked. Still, it's important to cook pork thoroughly to avoid food poisoning.

For safety as well as tenderness and flavor, cook pork

to the proper temperature so that you kill bacteria (such as *Salmonella*) as well as parasites that cause trichinosis and toxoplasmosis.

WILD GAME

Obviously, if you have a hunter in the family, the game he or she brings home won't have been state or federally inspected; parasites (*Trichinella spiralis* or *Toxoplasma gondii*) may have contaminated the meat, and improper handling in the field may have caused further contamination.

To cut down on problems, the hunter should dress the game in the field, right after shooting, and then chill as soon as possible (below 40°F) until it can be either cooked or frozen.

TAKEOUT

If you're buying ready-to-eat takeout meats (such as Chinese food, ribs, burgers, and so on), make sure the foods are hot when you buy them. Eat cooked meat within two hours (one hour on a hot day over 85°F) or refrigerate the product in shallow, covered containers at 40°F. If you refrigerate this food, use it up within three or four days; you can eat it cold or reheat to 165°F.

You can also freeze ready-to-serve meat dishes; use within four months for best quality.

6

Safe Seafood

High in protein, minerals, and cholesterol-lowering omega-3 fatty acids and low in calories, fat, and cholesterol, seafood is widely believed to be a very healthy source of nourishment. But it can also be a source of contamination and spoilage.

This is no small problem because in the past ten years Americans have begun eating much more fish than ever before—more than fifteen pounds per person annually. The problem is that fish readily soak up poisons and contaminants, concentrating heavy metals in their bodies, and shellfish pick up contaminants from the plankton they feed on in polluted water. Even in the cleanest waters, fish and shellfish meet up with naturally occurring marine bacteria, viruses, toxins, and pollutants. When contaminated fish are eaten by larger fish, the toxins are concentrated further. In big fish such as swordfish and tuna, the contaminants may reach levels harmful to humans.

The most common problems in seafood are scombroid

fish poisoning caused by spoilage, and ciguatera and paralytic shellfish poisoning, the result of naturally occurring toxic plankton.

SCOMBROID POISONING

Even under the best conditions, a fish keeps for only seven to twelve days; but it often takes seven days for the fish to get from the water to the supermarket, where it may sit for several more days. Scombroid decomposition, named for a particular suborder of marine bony fishes *(Scombroidei)*, is caused by poor handling on board fishing vessels, and by a toxic form of histamine that builds up quickly as fish lie in a boat at high temperatures. It's especially common in tuna, mackerel, mahimahi, bluefish, and albacore. Scombroid poisoning can cause immediate nausea, vomiting, and cramps; a tingling sensation around the mouth; rash; and abdominal pain, although symptoms subside after a day or two. You can tell your fish has scombroid decomposition if it has a peppery taste.

If you catch your own fish, you can prevent scombroid poisoning by making sure to chill and ice down your catch immediately after you pull it into the boat.

CIGUATERA POISONING

This food-borne illness is caused by microscopic toxic plankton found in warm waters of the Caribbean and off the coast of Hawaii that are eaten by game fish. There are thousands of cases each year. Ciguatera poisoning is very common in certain parts of the world; it occurs most often in the Caribbean islands, Florida and Hawaii, and the Pacific Islands. Recent reports revealed 129 cases over a two-year period in Dade County, Florida, alone. It appears to be occurring more often, probably because of the increased demand for seafood around the world. Experts believe this type of poisoning is underreported because it is usually not fatal and symptoms don't last long.

Isolated instances of ciguatera poisoning have occurred along the eastern United States coast, from South Florida to New Hampshire. The U.S. Virgin Islands and Puerto Rico also report sporadic cases. In this country it's more of a problem for sport fishermen, not restaurant patrons. Restaurants in areas where the toxin is common are careful not to serve tainted fish, so sport fishermen who eat their own catch run a much higher risk.

For information on a new kit that detects cigua toxin in fish, see Appendix B, "For More Information . . .".

BACTERIAL CONTAMINATION

Because bacteria that live in fish are adapted to withstand the cold waters of lakes and oceans, they can thrive in temperatures cold enough to preserve other food. These microbes will quickly spoil fish, unless it is kept at temperatures close to freezing.

Moreover, dangerous types of *E. coli* from feces can contaminate fish during handling anywhere along the line—boats, trucks, piers, processing plants, and fish markets. No matter how carefully fish are gutted and

What's in Your Seafood?

Seafood can be a very healthful food choice, but it also carries some risk. Here's a list of possible contamination or poison dangers for each type:

Amberjack	Cigua toxin
Bluefish	Scombroid toxin; PCBs
Clams	Shellfish poisoning
Cockles	Shellfish poisoning
Crabs	Shellfish poisoning
Grouper	Cigua toxin
Mackerel	Scombroid toxin
Oysters	*Salmonella,* hepatitis A, cholera, lead contamination, shellfish poisoning
Salmon	*Salmonella*; PCBs
Sea bass	Cigua toxin

Shellfish (all types)	Shellfish poisoning
Snapper	Cigua toxin
Surgeonfish	Cigua toxin
Sushi (raw fish)	*Anisakis* infection
Triggerfish	Cigua toxin
Tuna	Scombroid toxin; cadmium or mercury contamination

covered in ice on a boat, when they're thrown onto a pier covered with animal droppings and filth from people's shoes, and then left lying on the pier, bacteria can thrive.

CHEMICAL AND METALLIC RESIDUES

According to a 1991 report by the National Academy of Science, chemical residues were found in lakes, rivers, and coastal waters across the country. In 1992, *Consumer Reports* magazine discovered residues of the banned pesticide DDT in catfish and mercury in swordfish from New York and Chicago. It also discovered lead-contaminated clams and birth defect–causing PCBs in whitefish and salmon. Because these contaminants accumulate in our bodies, even low levels could be a serious problem over time.

Chlorinated Compounds

Fatty fish like salmon, bluefish, and herring are vulnerable to chlorinated compounds, such as PCBs (polychlorinated biphenyls) and the insecticide DDT, which linger in the body for years. Very minute quantities of these substances in the water will produce very high concentrations in fish. And because fish like striped bass and bluefish migrate, they can have high contamination levels no matter where they're caught.

Mercury

One of the most insidious types of mercury poisoning occurs through the contamination of fish in lakes and streams throughout the United States as a result of extensive agricultural fungicide and pesticide use, and the industrial by-products of chlorine production. Current estimates suggest that up to 10,000 tons of mercury infiltrate the sea each year; once in the water, the mercury enters the food chain, where it is converted into organic methyl mercury, one of the most toxic substances known to man.

The presence of sewage in the water facilitates this deadly conversion through bacteria living in the mud; once the conversion occurs, the contaminated bacteria are then eaten by plankton, which are in turn eaten by pike, pickerel, perch, walleye, muskie, and white bass.

Unlike inorganic mercury compounds, methyl mercury is hard to detect in the blood. It does not readily break down in the body and can take months to be excreted. In addition, it can pass easily through the blood-brain barrier, irreversibly damaging brain cells; it also crosses the placenta and builds up in the fetal brain and blood. Methyl mercury seems to affect women more than men, and it affects children and infants most of all.

The FDA mandates that tuna must contain less than 0.5 mg/kg of mercury. Scientists estimate that to be safe, humans should ingest no more than 0.1 mg of mercury per day; if a fish contains 1 part per billion of mercury, than the safe weekly limit would be about one portion of fish a week.

Unfortunately, very little is known about ways to remove the methyl mercury pollutants from contaminated water, which may remain poisoned for between ten and one hundred years. Pregnant women, nursing mothers, and young children should limit consumption of fish that might have high levels of mercury and PCBs to no more than once a month.

SHELLFISH

The problems of fish contamination and spoilage are not the only ones in the seafood industry: shellfish are also a source of food-borne illness. Shellfish are highly susceptible to bacterial and viral contamination, since they live close to the shore where pollution tends to be worse.

The most common way shellfish become tainted is by eating toxic plankton that multiply rapidly during the warm summer months; because the plankton have a pink or red color, this phenomenon has come to be called red tide.

Red Tide

Red tides are found in coastal waters (since waters offshore are not favorable to the growth of these plankton) in the Pacific from California to Alaska, in the Atlantic from New England up to the St. Lawrence, and along the west coast of Europe.

These plankton produce the deadly poison saxitoxin, which blocks nerve impulses and causes paralytic shellfish poisoning (PSP), and is so toxic that even one contaminated shellfish can be fatal if eaten. This is why clams, oysters, and mussels are not sold during months without an "R" (the summer months, when red tides occur).

Red tides have been known since ancient times; it is

believed that the Red Sea was named by ancient Greeks who were referring to red blooms off the Arabian coasts. The first reference to red tide is said to appear in the Bible: "And all the waters that were in the river were turned to blood. And the fish that was in the river died, and the river stank, and the Egyptians could not drink of the water of the rivers" (Exodus 7:20–21).

Mussels, clams, and oysters are the shellfish most at risk, and mussels most of all. Healthy bivalve shellfish filter large amounts of toxic plankton, which form the primary ocean food from May through August. During these warm times, the plankton thrive and can be so invasive that they kill birds and fish.

The first large epidemic of poisoning caused by shellfish contaminated by red tide occurred in San Francisco in 1927, when 102 people were sickened, and 6 died. Today, largely because of the prohibition against eating certain shellfish during the summer, such epidemics are rare.

Most cases of shellfish poisoning have occurred when people ate raw shellfish; cooking will kill bacteria (although heat must be very high to kill the hepatitis A virus). But nothing will eliminate the toxins that cause PSP. In addition to PSP, other types of shellfish poisoning include neurotoxic, diarrhetic, and amnesic shellfish poisoning.

Problems with shellfish contamination—and with the integrity of the seafood industry—have led to a number of incidents. Recent outbreaks of illness and death have prompted several states (including Florida, Louisiana, and California) to require that warning

Signs of Seafood Poisoning

Symptoms	Source	Onset
Stomach problems, hot and cold reversal, weakness, facial pain, numbness, headache, weakness	Red snapper, grouper, barracuda (ciguatera)	1–6 hours
Tingling/burning mouth; wheezing, rash, headaches, dropping blood pressure; nausea/vomiting; diarrhea	Tuna, mahimahi, mackerel, abalone, bluefish, sardines (scombroid)	Immediate–30 minutes
Stomach problems, memory loss, confusion, seizures, disorientation, coma	Mussels (neurotoxic, amnesic shellfish poisoning)	Within 6 hours

Symptoms	Source	Onset
Gradual paralysis, trembling, nausea/vomiting, diarrhea; shortness of breath; choking or slurred speech; lack of coordination	Mussels, clams (paralytic shellfish poisoning)	Within 30 minutes
Vomiting, twitching, weakness, respiratory paralysis	California newt, puffer fish, sunfish (tetrodotoxin)	30–40 minutes
Fever, fatigue, weakness, stomach problems, appetite loss, jaundice	Oysters/other shellfish (hepatitis A)	15–50 days
Fever, weakness, appetite loss, headache, diarrhea, nausea/vomiting, stomach pain	Shellfish (Norwalk virus)	1–2 days

notices be posted wherever raw shellfish is sold, detailing the risk of raw seafood in people with liver, stomach, blood, or immune disorders. Many state shellfish screening programs test shellfish for the presence of these toxins and monitor the safety of shellfish harvest beds. However, people who catch their own shellfish from unapproved beds are at risk for a variety of toxic infections.

Overall, your risk of getting sick from seafood is only about one in 250,000, according to the FDA. But public watchdog groups like the Public Voice for Food and Health Policy in Washington warn that government estimates may be misleading, since very few seafood-related illnesses are ever reported. Symptoms are so similar to other food-borne illnesses that many people—including doctors—can't tell the difference.

Bacterial and Viral Contamination in Shellfish

While shellfish by themselves are not poisonous, they can become contaminated by bacteria or viruses from their environment, then pass infection on up the food chain to humans. Oysters, clams, and mussels are particularly prone to contamination because of their respiratory systems, which pump water across their gills and isolate plankton, making these bivalves vulnerable to bacteria, viruses, and contaminants in the water. (Lobsters and other crustacean shellfish only rarely become contaminated.)

The most common cause of viral contamination in shellfish is the Norwalk virus, which can cause food poisoning when raw or improperly cooked food has been in contact with water contaminated by human excrement. *Vibrio* is another potential problem.

It's also possible to contract hepatitis A from eating raw shellfish harvested from sewage-contaminated waters.

Even though federal regulations and posting of contaminated waters offer some protection, there is still a risk of contracting viruses when eating raw shellfish.

WHAT YOU CAN DO

While we expect the government to watch out for food-borne illness problems, there is still a great deal we can do ourselves when buying, preparing, cooking, and serving seafood. When buying seafood, make sure you shop at a reputable dealer with a known record of safe handling practices. Avoid roadside stands. When looking for fish, observe how the store displays the product.

Safe Displays

Once the fish arrives at the market, there are further opportunities for spoilage. If raw fish are displayed in piles, the ones on the top often get warmer than the recommended 40°F. As bacteria multiply, the juices may be trickling down to fish underneath, spreading contamination. Displaying cooked and raw fish together can also be hazardous. While packaging can protect fish from cross-contamination, it also insulates fish from the cold, and when packages are stacked, the ones on top are even more likely to begin to deteriorate from the heat.

Choosing Seafood

Choose a fish from the bottom of the refrigerator case, where it is coldest. Look at the fish you're going to buy: it should look and smell fresh and have no fishy or ammonia odor. Its eyes should be fresh-looking, not cloudy or sunken, and it should be a good color, with bright pink or red gills.

Lobsters, crabs, clams, and oysters are best when bought alive and cooked at home. Choose only live mollusks (their shells are tightly shut; that is, they won't move when pinched). Discard any clams or oysters whose shells are cracked.

Fresh or Frozen?

At the seafood counter, the word "fresh" is supposed to mean never frozen or heated. "Fresh frozen" on the label indicates the seafood was frozen when it was fresh, often within hours of harvest. If fish products were frozen and thawed for retail sale, they should be labeled "previously frozen."

In the Cart

Once you've bought your seafood, pack it separately in the bags, or put it on top of the grocery bags. Seafood won't last long in a hot car on a long drive home. If you're buying seafood at the supermarket, make it one of your very last purchases. If will take more than an hour to reach your house from the store, bring a cooler along to store the seafood.

STORAGE AT HOME

Once you get your seafood home, how long you can safely keep it depends on how well you take care of it, and whether it's a whole fish or a live mollusk. You should keep your seafood very cold and eat it within one or two days. Store seafood in the original wrapper in the coldest part (usually the meat drawer) of the refrigerator; temperature should be as close to 32°F as possible. (Many home refrigerators maintain temperature at 40°F; at this temperature, storage time is limited.)

Fish

Because fish bruises easily, be sure to use both hands to lift the piece and not to pick it up by the tail. If you have dressed fish, pack it on ice. Fillets and steaks should be in plastic bags or containers; cover with ice in trays or pans. Empty melt-water regularly and add more ice as necessary.

If the fish isn't prepackaged, wash it under cold, running water and pat dry with an absorbent paper towel. Then wrap the fish in moisture-proof paper or plastic wrap, put it in a plastic bag, or store it in an airtight rigid container until you are ready to cook.

Shellfish

The way you handle and store the shellfish depends on the variety of shellfish that you buy. Live shellfish should be kept in a shallow container covered with moist cloths or a moistened paper towel—not in an airtight bag or container, where they could die. Don't store in water. However, a few hours before steaming, you can submerge clams in cold salt water (add some cornmeal to help the clams spit out sand). Change the water several times in order to reduce the amount of grit in the clams.

Remember to avoid cross-contamination in your refrigerator. Keep juices from raw seafood away from all other food. Store shrimp, squid, and shucked shellfish in a leakproof bag, plastic container, or covered jar.

Follow these storage time limits to make sure your seafood is safe:

- Use squid and fresh-shucked clams within one or two days.
- Use shrimp and scallops within two or three days.
- Use fresh-shucked oysters within five to seven days.
- Use live lobsters and crabs the same day they are bought.
- Use live mussels and clams in the shell within two to three days; use oysters in the shell within seven to ten days. If the shells have opened during storage, tap them. The shells should close—throw away those that don't.
- Use cooked, whole lobsters or crabs within two to three days.
- You can store cooked, picked lobster or crabmeat in the refrigerator in a sealed moisture-proof plastic bag or airtight plastic container for three to four days.
- You can store pasteurized crabmeat in the refrigerator for up to six months before opening.

DEFROSTING

You don't always have to defrost seafood before cooking, depending on how you're going to be cooking it. If you aren't going to defrost before cooking, double the cooking time. If you intend to coat, roll, or stuff the fish, you'll need to defrost it so that you can handle it easily.

If you have time, try to defrost fish overnight in the refrigerator; this will minimize the loss of moisture. A one-pound package will defrost within twenty-four hours. Thaw frozen seafood in the refrigerator on a plate to catch the juices; don't let the juices drip onto anything else in the refrigerator. *Never defrost seafood at room temperature, or in a warm- or hot-water bath.*

PREPARING

Just before cooking, scrub live oysters, clams, and mussels with a stiff vegetable brush. If you're preparing seafood for later use, refrigerate or freeze immediately in shallow containers after cooking. Don't worry about adding a warm seafood dish to the refrigerator or freezer; modern appliances are designed to compensate for a few temporarily hot foods without allowing other foods to warm up.

When you're finished preparing the seafood, wash the cutting board, utensils, counter, sink, and your hands with hot, soapy water, and use a fingernail brush to clean your cuticles and under your nails. Be sure your sponges and dishcloths are clean.

COOKING

Fish

Cook fin fish thoroughly, using the "10-minute rule"—allow 10 minutes per one-inch thickness whether baking, broiling, poaching, frying, barbecuing, or stewing. Measure the fish at its thickest point (if the fish is to be stuffed or rolled, measure it after stuffing or rolling). Turn the fish when it's halfway through the cooking time. (Pieces of fish less than a half-inch thick don't have to be turned over.)

If you're cooking the fish in foil, or in a sauce, add another 5 minutes to the total cooking time. Double the cooking time for fish that hasn't been defrosted. Fish is cooked when it begins to flake and loses its raw appearance; it should reach an internal temperature of 145°F. Avoid interrupted cooking; cook fish and shellfish fully at one time—partial cooking can encourage bacterial growth.

Don't taste seafood while it's cooking.

If you're cooking fillets, broil them on a rack and let the juices drip out; if you discard these drippings, you can greatly lower the concentration of pesticides and chemical and metallic residues (but not mercury). Because pesticides concentrate in fatty tissue, trim and throw away the skin and fat portions from the top, side, and belly of fish at risk for contaminants (such as Great Lakes fish).

Guarding Against Contaminants

Although it's important to cook seafood thoroughly, remember that no amount of cooking will destroy contaminants. If you have reason to worry about chemical or metallic residues, scrape off the fatty skin before cooking. Pregnant women, nursing mothers, and young children should not eat too much fish that might have high levels of mercury and PCBs. The healthiest type of fish to eat are low-fat fish caught far offshore. Haddock may be your best bet, with the lowest levels of PCBs and pesticides.

Shellfish

While it's important to cook shellfish long enough, it's also important not to overcook them, because then the meat will be tough, dry, and flavorless. Some shellfish are already cooked when you buy them (canned clams, picked crabmeat, and artificial surimi products). In this case, all you have to do is to heat the precooked shellfish or surimi to the desired temperature without cooking further.

Shrimp and Scallops

It takes from 3 to 5 minutes to boil or steam a pound of medium shrimp, and from 3 to 4 minutes to cook scallops. They will be firm and opaque when done.

Shucked Shellfish

Clams, mussels, and oysters are plump and opaque when cooked completely. The FDA recommends that you:

- boil or simmer shucked oysters at least 3 minutes
- fry shucked oysters in oil at least 10 minutes at 375°F
- bake shellfish at 450°F for at least 10 minutes

Steaming Shellfish

When steaming shellfish, use small pots. If you cook too many at once, you may not be able to cook the centers thoroughly. Experts recommend the following steaming times for shellfish:

- Clams, mussels, and oysters: in the shell for 4 to 9 minutes from the start of steaming. Discard any oysters, clams, or mussels whose shells don't open during cooking, since the closed shell suggests the mollusk may not have been heated enough.
- Lobsters: 10 to 12 minutes per pound, starting from when the water returns to a boil. Boiled lobsters and steamed crabs turn bright red.
- Crabs: (two to three dozen) for 25 minutes (depending on size) in a large crab pot.

Microwaving Seafood

Microwaving seafood can be a very healthy, tasty way of preparing it—provided you follow the rules for safe cooking. While microwaving heats the surface of the food quickly, it's important to allow enough time for the waves to penetrate to the center of the food.

When you microwave, remember to cover the food to hold in moisture and make sure the food cooks evenly. Use a microwave-safe dish, or cover the food with waxed paper when microwaving. Plastic wrap can cover a container but shouldn't touch the food. Use a turntable when cooking in a microwave; if you don't have one, turn the entire dish several times during cooking. Always stir food when possible at least twice during cooking. After you finish cooking the seafood, allow it to stand for the recommended time in the recipe to complete the cooking process. Check for doneness before serving.

EATING IT RAW: YES OR NO?

Since cooking can destroy most harmful organisms in seafood, simply giving up raw seafood can significantly cut your risk. Raw clams, oysters, and other shellfish are linked to nearly one thousand cases of hepatitis A alone each year. Other food-borne illnesses you can get include cholera, salmonellosis, listeriosis, and a wide variety of parasites. People with liver problems, the very young, the very old, and anyone with a chronic illness or impaired immune system should never eat raw seafood at all.

Still not convinced? If you insist on eating raw seafood, eat it only during the cold months when there is less chance of toxic organisms being present. Go to a raw bar where you can watch them open the shellfish in front of you.

Aficionados of raw seafood also frequent sushi bars, the Japanese restaurants that specialize in serving raw seafood. Many people love sushi and willingly accept the risk of food-borne illness, primarily parasites that aren't usually deadly unless you are at high risk.

If you're going to eat raw seafood anyway, you may want to avoid pike, perch, or salmon, together with the saltwater fish such as European herring, mackerel, rockfish, squid, cod, whiting, and haddock. You should be particularly careful with raw Pacific salmon. Remember

Safer Sushi Choices

If you love sushi, you'll be happy to know that the most common types of fish used very rarely harbor parasites. These include:

- tuna (bluefin, yellowfin, and albacore or *shiro maguro*)
- Japanese yellowtail (young, *hamachi*)
- fish roe (other than herring roe)
- octopus
- shrimp
- scallops

Worst Picks

These types of sushi are probably least safe:

- herring roe (*kazunoki*)
- mackerel (*saba*)
- salmon (*sake*)
- freshwater fish

that parasites can survive even a dunking in lime juice as part of the preparation for seviche. And neither soaking in vinegar nor salting destroys the *Anisakis* parasite.

LEFTOVERS

Taking care of leftovers is an extremely important part of food safety, particularly when it comes to seafood. This is often where people make mistakes. To prevent a problem, wash hands before handling leftovers. Use clean utensils and surfaces. Refrigerate or freeze leftovers in covered shallow containers within two hours after cooking. Be sure to leave air space around the containers to allow circulation of cold air, and to be sure the food cools evenly. Date leftovers so you know how long they've been in storage.

Before serving, cover and reheat leftovers to 160°F. Soups, sauces, and other leftover liquids should be reheated to a rolling boil.

Once you've opened pasteurized crabmeat, use within three to five days. If you open canned fish (such as tuna or salmon), store leftovers in a glass or plastic container in the refrigerator.

CATCHING IT YOURSELF

Fish

If you're going to be catching—and eating—your own fish, there are some rules to follow to make sure the fish is as safe as possible.

First, scale, gut, and clean the fish as soon as they're caught. Wrap them in watertight plastic, and store on ice in a cooler, with three to four inches of ice in the bottom. Alternate layers of fish and layers of ice, and keep the cooler out of direct sunlight. Cover it with a tarp or other covering if you can.

Once you get your fish home, plan to eat them within a day or two, or freeze the catch. If you freeze it, you'll want to eat it within six months for best flavor.

Shellfish

When you go hunting for shellfish, remember that you've got to keep your catch alive until you cook it. Store the shellfish in live wells, or out of water in a bushel or other container covered with wet burlap.

Follow these rules for safe eating:

- Crabs or lobsters: eat the same day they're caught.
- Live oysters: eat within 7 to 10 days.
- Mussels and clams: eat within 4 to 5 days.

WHAT THE GOVERNMENT IS DOING

In the past, the seafood industry was not tightly regulated by the federal government. The FDA was responsible for monitoring fish safety only by inspecting the seafood processors, and budget and staff constraints hampered even these minimum efforts. Fishing boats weren't inspected at all, and markets were monitored by understaffed and overworked state and local agencies.

Because of growing concerns over seafood safety,

the FDA established a state-of-the-art safety program called the Hazard Analysis Critical Control Points (HACCP) that focuses on the parts of the processing system where contamination is most likely. Developed in 1959 to ensure the strictest safety standards for food eaten by astronauts, it is now used throughout the country in the seafood industry.

HACCP targets both fresh and processed seafood, and features a self-monitoring system where individual plants keep logs of storage temperatures, equipment cleaning schedules, and storage dates. FDA agents visit the plants for routine inspections and check the books for errors.

The program is supported by the seafood industry, the National Academy of Science, and most consumer groups. Processors and packers complied with the new regulations in 1995. The rules were implemented on trawlers as well as at fish-processing facilities, retail markets, and restaurants.

While there won't be any changes in the way seafood is packaged, labeled, or displayed, the program is designed to improve consumers' confidence in seafood.

7

The Chicken or the Egg: How to Protect Your Family

What could be more American than a couple of sunny-side up eggs or a bucket of fried chicken? And yet poultry products carry one of the highest known risks of food poisoning: *Salmonella,* the most frequently reported cause of food-borne illness.

Each year the Centers for Disease Control and Prevention document about 40,000 cases of salmonellosis—and those are the ones that get reported. But poultry also carries other potential food-borne infections as well. Chickens can be infected with *Campylobacter jejuni* bacteria (it is estimated that one-third to one-half of all raw chicken on the market is contaminated). *Campylobacter* infections strike between 2 million and 4 million Americans each year.

CONTROLLING INFECTION

Salmonella is carried mostly in the digestive tracts of healthy birds on chicken farms, where the problem may spread undetected among the flocks. Some experts suspect that *Campylobacter* in poultry may be spread through contaminated drinking water. Since most of the known cases of contaminated poultry occur in large poultry operations and plants, it is unclear if smaller operations have less of a problem. For example, experts don't know if kosher chickens or free-range chickens are lower in bacteria than chickens from large operations.

When the birds are slaughtered, bacteria are transferred from the intestines to the meat. As they currently operate, chicken processing plants appear to be the primary contributors to *Salmonella* and *Campylobacter* contamination: bacteria can breed in the water baths designed to loosen feathers, and the microorganisms are then pounded into the skin by defeathering machines. Carcasses that are eviscerated by machine can be contaminated by fecal matter. Processing plants use chlorine washes and chilly temperatures to control the bacteria, but poor quality control at some plants means that the bacteria still wind up on between 20 and 60 percent of chickens in the grocery stores. Bone meal, fertilizer, and pet foods as well as poultry for human consumption may all be implicated in the spread of salmonellosis.

Salmonella may also contaminate cracked or broken eggs, and it can even be found in intact eggs if an infected chicken passes on the bacteria directly to the eggs still in her ovaries. While the chance of finding a salmonella-contaminated egg is small (only 1 in 20,000), the USDA recommends that everyone avoid eating foods and beverages made with raw eggs (such as hollandaise sauce or eggnog).

WHAT YOU CAN DO

Part of the battle against these bacteria is still up to us, since proper handling and cooking can eliminate bacterial contamination in eggs and poultry. There are many things you can do to protect yourself and your family from getting sick from salmonellosis and campylobacteriosis.

IN THE SUPERMARKET

Poultry
When you're shopping, pick up fresh chickens, turkeys, ducks, and geese last, and check the "sell by" date. Store poultry in your cart away from other food. Some people carry plastic bags to put packages of chicken into, since the plastic trays of chicken parts can leak potentially contaminated juice. Once at the checkout counter, insist that the poultry products be bagged separately.

Giblets
Giblets are the heart, liver, and gizzard of poultry; they're often simmered to make gravy, or used in

appetizers and main dishes. (Although often packaged with them, the neck of a bird is not a giblet.)

There are no grading standards for giblets. In whole, ready-to-cook poultry, giblets are included in a paper bag in the abdominal cavity. However, the giblets packed in the bird are not those from the same bird. Ready-to-cook poultry products aren't required to contain giblets, but if a bird is labeled as "with giblets" it must contain at least half of each giblet from a bird. If you wish, you can also buy giblets separately, as livers, hearts, or a combination.

How can you tell whether your giblets are of good quality? Normal poultry liver may be any color from tan to yellow or deep red; a yellow liver indicates high fat content, not disease. In fact, the color of a giblet depends on what the bird ate last, and has nothing to do with age or health.

Sometimes you may notice that a liver looks a bit green; the coloring is caused by bile that leaches out of the gallbladder and into the liver. Normally, green livers are removed at the slaughter plant and not sold to the public because they don't look very attractive, but they won't hurt you if one slips by and you eat it. Or you may notice that the gallbladder or portion of it is still attached to the liver (it looks like a little green pill). The gallbladder is generally removed, but sometimes it's missed at the plant. You can remove the gallbladder yourself, and then eat the liver.

When buying giblets, select them just before checking out at the register; the giblets should feel cold to the touch. Giblets aren't required to be dated, but many stores voluntarily date packages of giblets and poultry with giblets. Check the "sell by" date. You should use or freeze giblets within a day or two of purchase. If there is a "use by" date, observe it. (The "use by" date is for quality assurance; after the date, peak quality begins to drop, but the product may still be used. Always try to buy a product before the "use by" date.)

Place giblets in a disposable plastic bag if possible to trap any potential leakage that might contaminate other food.

Eggs

Always buy Grade A or AA eggs with clean, uncracked shells from a refrigerated display case. Do not buy eggs anywhere where they aren't refrigerated. Any bacteria in the egg can quickly grow at room temperature. Take eggs directly home.

STORAGE AT HOME

When you're putting food away in the refrigerator at home, put packages of chicken on a tray or plate to catch dripping juices. Store at 40°F (or colder) in your refrigerator and use within a day or two. If you aren't going to be using the chicken by that time, freeze it at 0°F in its original packaging.

Giblets

Immediately place in the refrigerator any separate giblets you have bought and use within a day or two, or freeze at 0°F. If kept frozen, they will keep indefinitely, but for best quality you should use them within three or four months.

Poultry Leftovers

Don't let stuffed poultry stand unrefrigerated for long periods. However, you should never refrigerate a whole cooked large bird (such as a turkey); it can take too long to cool down to a safe temperature. Instead, cut meat off the bone and refrigerate (drumsticks, legs, and wings may be kept whole). Remove the stuffing after cooking and promptly refrigerate it.

Eggs

Place eggs in their original grocery carton in the coldest part of the refrigerator. (Don't store on the door; it's not cold enough.) Don't wash the eggs before storing.

If any eggs have cracked on the ride home—and you know they were uncracked when you bought them—you can break those eggs into a clean container, cover tightly, and keep refrigerated for use within two days.

Use refrigerated intact raw eggs within three to five weeks. Once they're hard-boiled, eggs will keep in the refrigerator for up to a week. Leftover yolks and whites should be used within two to four days after you break the shell.

You can't freeze fresh raw or hard-boiled eggs in the shell, but you can freeze raw yolks or whites, either separated or blended, for up to a year. To freeze whole eggs out of the shell, beat yolks and whites together (egg whites can also be frozen by themselves) and use within a year.

If your eggs accidentally freeze in their shells, go ahead and keep them frozen until needed. Defrost them in the refrigerator, and discard any with cracked shells.

Avoid keeping eggs outside the refrigerator for more than two hours (or a shorter time in a hot kitchen in the summer). Don't leave hard-boiled and decorated Easter eggs in the Easter baskets for long periods of time.

Dishes made with eggs may be refrigerated for later use (within three to four days). Leftovers should be divided into shallow containers for quick cooling and placed in the refrigerator.

DEFROSTING

Never defrost poultry on the counter; instead, place the wrapped bird in the fridge. Or you can immerse it in a bowl of cold water that you then change every half hour. A whole 3- to 4-pound fryer with giblets should thaw in two to three hours with this method; a whole 15-pound turkey will take seven to eight hours (or about 30 minutes a pound). A one-pound carton of frozen chicken livers will thaw in one or two hours with this method.

When defrosting giblets, it's best to plan on a slow, safe thaw in the refrigerator. Normally, a whole bird with giblets will take about twenty-four hours for every 5 pounds of weight. A 1-pound carton of frozen chicken livers will take about twenty-four hours to defrost. Once defrosted, giblets can be stored in the refrigerator for a day or two. After this, if the giblets haven't been used, you can refreeze them safely.

If you choose to defrost giblets in a cold-water bath, leave them in their original airtight package or place in a leak-proof plastic bag. Change the water every 30 minutes.

If microwave-defrosting, plan to cook the bird immediately after thawing.

While you can refreeze food defrosted in the refrigerator, foods defrosted in the microwave or in cold water should be cooked before refreezing.

PREPARING

Because many types of food poisoning are spread by the fecal-oral route, it's vitally important that you wash your hands after using the toilet and before preparing food. Anyone with diarrhea and/or vomiting should use a separate towel and washcloth and should not prepare food (especially uncooked food).

Cut the poultry on a nonporous cutting board of plastic or acrylic that is dishwasher safe, so you can sanitize it between uses. Some people like to reserve one board solely for use with poultry and meats, and use another for vegetables and fruits, and another for bread.

If you're going to marinate the poultry, do so in the refrigerator—not out in room temperature. You can marinate chicken, duck, or goose in the fridge for up to two days.

After you handle the raw poultry, be sure to wash your hands and anything else that touched it—utensils, cutting board, sink, counters, etc.—with hot, soapy water.

COOKING

Be sure to cook your poultry to an internal temperature high enough to kill harmful bacteria. For tenderness and doneness, the USDA recommends cooking whole poultry to 180°F. Use an instant-read thermometer that you insert into the thickest part of the bird—be sure not to let it touch bone. It's not safe to partially cook poultry or to microwave whole stuffed poultry. The meat will cook so fast that the stuffing inside might not reach a hot enough temperature.

Don't cook a large bird (such as turkey) overnight in a slow oven; poultry should never be cooked in an oven set lower than 325°F.

If you cook poultry pieces in a microwave, remember that microwave ovens vary in power and efficiency. Check the pieces in several places to make sure of the temperature and doneness.

Cooked muscle meats can be pink even when the meat has reached a safe internal temperature. If fresh poultry has reached 180°F throughout the meat, it should be safe to eat even if it's still pink in the middle. The pink color may be due to the cooking method, or ingredients that you've added later. Many consumers have been conditioned to be wary of the pink color in pork, and so when they see other meats with that rosy appearance, red warning flags pop up in their minds. The color of cooked meat and poultry isn't always a sure sign of its doneness. Only by using a meat thermometer can you really determine when the meat has reached a safe temperature. Turkey may still be pink after cooking to temperatures of 160°F or higher, and the meat of smoked turkey is always pink. In general, poultry meat is lighter in color than beef because poultry has much less pigment. As the bird ages, this pigment level usually increases.

Giblets

Most people cook giblets by simmering them in water for use in flavoring soups, gravies, or stuffing. Once cooked, the liver becomes crumbly, and the heart and gizzard soften and are easy to chop. The juices of cooked giblets should run clear. Casseroles containing giblets should be cooked to 160°F; stuffing should be cooked to 165°F.

When giblets come paper-wrapped inside the bird's body, people sometimes inadvertently cook them inside the bird still wrapped. The giblets are safe to eat when cooked by mistake this way (although it's not recommended), as long as they are cooked to a safe temperature.

However, if giblets are packed in a plastic bag and the bag has melted or changed shape during the cooking process, you should discard both giblets and poultry, since harmful chemicals may have leached into the surrounding meat. If the plastic bag has not changed during cooking, the giblets and poultry should be safe to use as long as the meat is fully cooked.

Ground Poultry

While everybody is familiar with ground beef, some consumers may not realize it's also possible to buy

Safe Internal Temperature

Poultry is safe to eat if the internal temperature is:

- whole bird: 180°F
- bone-in breast: 170°F
- bone-in thigh: 180°F
- ground poultry: 165°F
- stuffing (in bird): 165°F
- whole boneless parts: 160°F

ground poultry, which is commonly found in the fresh or frozen meat case at your grocery store.

There are no established regulatory standards for ground poultry, and producers aren't required to identify on the label what cuts of poultry they have ground up. However, there are these basic guidelines: Ground poultry can contain only muscle meat and skin with attached fat, without other components (such as giblets). While the federal government encourages voluntary nutrition labeling on ground poultry products, it doesn't require it.

When you cook ground poultry, you should always make sure the product reaches an internal temperature of 165°F; leftovers should be reheated to 165°F.

Smoked Poultry

It's important to remember that poultry is smoked for flavor, not preservation. If a smoked poultry product is labeled "keep refrigerated," that's a warning it needs to be refrigerated and kept cold to be safe to eat. Follow the same storage procedures as you would for other types of raw poultry.

Ducks and Geese

When we think of poultry, most folks imagine chicken, but there are also a fair number of ducks and geese sold in grocery stores—especially around holiday time. Unfortunately, chicken isn't the only type of poultry that can be contaminated with bacteria; ducks and geese are also possible sources of infection.

Almost all ducks are raised indoors to protect them

from predators, and most are raised in Wisconsin and Indiana. Geese are raised indoors for the first six weeks of their life, and then they are put out to graze on grass and grain.

No hormones are allowed in either goose or duck production in this country, and very few drugs have been approved for use with these birds. If an antibiotic is given to cure a disease, a "withdrawal" period is required from the time the drug is given until it is legal to slaughter. Additives aren't allowed either, although if the meat or giblets are processed (as in pâté), then additives like MSG may be used. These will be listed on the product label.

All ducks and geese are federally inspected, but grading is voluntary (a plant pays to have its poultry graded). Irradiation has not been approved for ducks or geese.

Because there is less demand for ducks and geese, you'll usually find these products in the frozen food case at your supermarket, although they may be available fresh during holidays.

When cooking geese and ducks, you should follow the same preparation standards and cooking temperatures as for chicken.

Ratites (Emu, Ostrich, Rhea)

Even more unusual but growing in favor is yet another type of poultry: the ratites, which are becoming very popular as a source of lean meat that tastes like beef but contains much less fat. (In fact, ratites have fewer calories than chicken and turkey.) This family of flightless birds is among the largest in the world, and includes emu, ostrich, and rhea. There are now about one thousand ostrich farmers in the United States, and about ten thousand families are raising emu in forty-three states. Rhea are the newest ratites to be raised in the United States and number about fifteen thousand birds.

Voluntary ostrich inspection has been available since 1991. Recently, a grant of inspection was approved by the USDA for all ratites. Businesses pay an hourly fee for voluntary inspection, which is done on a carcass-by-carcass basis. Ratite meat is sold as a steak, fillet, medallions, roast, or ground meat.

While they are poultry, ratites are classified as "red" meat, and they are actually very red—a dark cherry red. Because the ratites are classified as red meat, ratite steaks and roasts can be safely cooked to medium rare (145°F) or medium (160°F); ground ratite meat should be cooked to 160°F.

Eggs

Avoid eating raw or undercooked eggs. Limit foods that contain raw eggs, including:

- milkshakes
- Caesar salad
- hollandaise sauce
- homemade mayonnaise
- homemade ice cream
- eggnog

It's important to cook eggs long enough to kill any bacteria that may be present. People at high risk should eat only hard-boiled or firm eggs.

The USDA recommends:

- Fried eggs: cook for 2 to 3 minutes on each side (or 4 minutes total in a covered pan) until yolk thickens.
- Scrambled eggs: cook until firm (not runny) for at least 1 minute.
- Poached eggs: cook for 5 minutes over boiling water.
- Soft-boiled eggs: cook in the shell in boiling water for 7 minutes.

Egg Products

When most of us think of eggs, we tend to think of white or brown ovals. But in fact, more than 25 percent of the eggs eaten each year are in the form of "egg products."

Egg products include liquid, frozen, and dried eggs that are widely used by the food service industry and as ingredients in other foods, such as prepared mayonnaise and ice cream. Egg products are made from eggs that have been removed from their shells for processing. They are pasteurized, cooled, frozen or dried, and packaged. You can buy whole eggs, whites, yolks, and various blends, with or without non-egg ingredients. Officially inspected egg products bear the USDA inspection mark.

Certain foods are not considered to be "egg products"; these include freeze-dried products, imitation egg products, and egg substitutes.

Why would someone use egg products? Safety, for

one reason. If you have your heart set on recipes that formerly used raw eggs, you can still prepare your favorites using commercially prepared pasteurized eggs or egg substitutes, or start with a cooked egg base (such as cooked custard for homemade ice cream). You can use egg products in baking or cooking (e.g., for scrambled eggs).

Dried egg mix is a USDA-inspected blend of dried whole eggs, nonfat dry milk, soybean oil, and a small amount of salt; it is mixed with water to approximate fresh eggs. Dried egg mix is distributed by the USDA to food banks, Indian reservations, needy family outlets, and disaster relief operations.

TAKEOUT

If you're picking up a big basket of cooked chicken for dinner, be sure it's hot when you pick it up, and use it within two hours. If you can't use it that quickly, then cut it into several pieces and refrigerate in shallow covered containers. When you're ready to eat, you can serve it cold or reheat to 165°F so that it's hot and steamy.

WHAT THE GOVERNMENT IS DOING

As a result of rising bacterial contamination, the U.S. government has recently imposed stricter standards on poultry processors. Under the USDA's new science-based inspection system, the Food Safety and

For More Information

For details on the safe preparation and handling of poultry, shell eggs, and egg dishes, call the USDA Meat and Poultry Hotline at 800-535-4555, Monday through Friday from 10 A.M. to 4 P.M. EST.

Inspection Service tests poultry samples to identify pathogens (especially *Salmonella*). For the first time, the FSIS is requiring all plants to reduce bacteria by means of a Hazard Analysis and Critical Control Points plan. As of autumn 1998, the HACCP plan has cut in half the cases of salmonella in chickens.

Since 1994, the government has required mandatory nutrition labeling for most poultry products except raw, single-ingredient products such as raw chicken breasts or ground poultry. However, if a company uses a term such as "lean" to describe the product, then the company must include a nutrition label. Safe handling instructions were required as of 1994, providing those who handle food with critical information.

As of 1995, processed products (such as hot dogs) that include mechanically separated poultry must say so on their label. Mechanically separated poultry is produced by high-pressure machinery that separates bone from poultry skeletal muscle tissue by crushing the bone and then forcing bone and tissue through a screening device. The final cake of pastelike material is very different from other boneless poultry products.

In addition, a new treatment for poultry may prevent *Salmonella* bacteria in chickens by growing benign microbes inside newly hatched chicks. In 1998 the FDA approved the use of Preempt, a spray that seems to eliminate *Salmonella* in chicks with just one application. Preempt is sprayed on newly hatched chicks in a solution that contains twenty-nine different kinds of "good" bacteria. As the chicks peck at their wet feathers, they also ingest the solution; the "good" bacteria then multiply in the chicks' intestinal tracts, shutting out other microbes, including *Salmonella*. Since there isn't enough food for all the microbes, the "good" bacteria win. The spray mimics what once occurred naturally: chicks used to ingest benign bacteria through their mother's droppings. However, modern agricultural practices mean that most chicks never see their mothers, and therefore don't get these helpful bacteria the natural way.

Preempt marks the first time the FDA has ever approved a mix of bacteria as an animal drug. Experts hope that delivering a healthier bird to the processing plant will improve the safety of the food when it finally arrives in the grocery stores. Scientists are now studying whether the product also can prevent *Salmonella* from getting into eggs.

8

Fruits and Vegetables

Most people don't associate seemingly harmless fruits and vegetables with deadly food poisoning, but in fact there can be lots of bacteria hiding amid all those vitamins. After all, these foods are grown in soil, a rich source of microbes, and the water used to irrigate them can be polluted with manure and pesticides. Once harvested, produce can be tainted anywhere along the route from farm to fork: there are potential problems with storage and transportation, and poor handling by grocers, restaurants, and even the home cook.

Not long ago, a sixteen-month-old Colorado girl died and sixty-nine other people got sick from drinking unpasteurized apple juice contaminated with *E. coli* bacteria. There seem to be more and more cases of food poisoning associated with produce, in part because Americans are eating more fresh fruit and veggies—up nearly 50 percent since 1970.

There have been many examples of food-borne infection traceable to fresh fruits and vegetables: *Salmonella* in cantaloupes, hepatitis A in frozen strawberries, *E. coli*–tainted fresh apple cider, *Shigella* in tossed salad, *Cyclospora* in imported raspberries.

The Food and Drug Administration does try to regulate some aspects of fruit and vegetable production, banning the use of some animal fertilizers and allowing only unpolluted water for irrigation. These rules apply to U.S. growers who sell produce in states other than their own, and also to foreign producers who sell produce to this country. And Congress is considering legislation to require the FDA to halt the import of fruits and vegetables from countries where food safety standards fall below acceptable levels.

IMPORTED PRODUCE

As the U.S. government has opened the door to more and more food from abroad, it has also unwittingly opened the door to more food-borne illnesses from contaminated produce. There have been outbreaks linked to imported strawberries, lettuce, raspberries, basil, and other produce.

While the FDA has numerous regulations for U.S. growers, it has limited ability to regulate imported produce. Take pesticides, for example. Organochlorines such as DDT, aldrin, dieldrin, heptachlor, chlordane, and endrin are all illegal in this country, but they are used in other countries and come flooding back to the U.S. markets in coffee, Mexican tomatoes, basmati rice, chocolate, bananas, tea, sugar, and vegetables.

While the FDA reports it is finding high or illegal

levels of residues in less than 2 percent of the food it tests coming from other countries, the problem doesn't always originate in the farmers' fields. Chemicals added after harvest are considered additives, and aren't included in residue testing. For example, it's legal to spray insect-killing fumigants all over domestic and imported food before shipping.

A recent report by the U.S. General Accounting Office (GAO) finds the FDA's control of imported food to be inadequate, and calls for more authority over imports, especially since the number of imported foods has doubled in the last five years.

PESTICIDE CONTAMINATION

While not technically a cause of food-borne illness, possible pesticide contamination of fruits and vegetables has some consumers worried. The FDA maintains that the U.S. fruit and vegetable supply doesn't contain excessive pesticides and that the benefits of eating fresh produce are much stronger than any possible risk from residues.

However, if you're worried about pesticide contamination, there are ways you can minimize your risk.

First, wash fruits and vegetables with water. Most experts agree that washing, cooking, and freezing dilute or degrade a high percentage of harmful residues. If you're going to be eating the outer skin of the item (such as an apple, cucumber, or potato) scrub with a brush (when appropriate). Throw away the outer leaves of leafy vegetables. When appropriate, you can peel and cook the vegetables and fruits, although you may lose some nutrients this way.

Most pesticides begin breaking down with exposure to sun, rain, and other elements soon after they are applied, and are usually below tolerance levels before leaving the farm.

To reduce the danger from pesticide-contaminated food, try to buy organic produce that has been grown without the use of pesticides. Look for the certification labels from organic farming associations (such as the California Certified Organic Farmers or the Organic Foods Production Association of North America).

AFLATOXINS

If you've ever bought a bag of peanuts from a bin at the grocery store, you've risked excessive levels of mold and its toxins. It's estimated that one of the most widespread of the toxins is aflatoxin, found in a wide variety of foods, including nuts (especially peanuts). Aflatoxin is a cancer-causing by-product of the *Aspergillus flavus* mold, which grows on peanuts, corn, wheat, rice, cottonseed, barley, soybeans, Brazil nuts, and pistachios. The mold that produces aflatoxin flourishes in warm, humid climates in the southeastern United States, but the mold can also appear elsewhere when rain falls on corn or wheat that is left in the field to dry. Aflatoxin-producing mold can even grow on plants damaged by insects or drought, poor nutrition or

Foods Least Likely
to Have Pesticide Contamination

The following foods have been found to contain the lowest number of detectable pesticides and chemical residues.

asparagus	corn	onions
avocados	dates	oranges
bananas	figs	papayas
beets	garlic	peas
brussels sprouts	grapefruit	pineapple
cabbage	green beans	tangerines
carrots	leeks	watercress
cauliflower	lemons	watermelon
coconut	limes	yams

unseasonable temperatures. The way agricultural products are stored can affect the mold's growth, but
the length of time of such storage is also important: the
longer agricultural products are stored in bins, the
greater the chance that environmental conditions favorable to aflatoxin production will be created. Stored nuts
or seeds might accidentally get wet or the storage bin
might not facilitate drying quickly enough to stop the
mold from growing.

Still, scientists know very little about why or how
the mold produces aflatoxin, and because the mold is
sometimes difficult to see, all susceptible crops are subject to routine testing in the United States. Unfortunately, it is not possible to detect the mold with 100
percent accuracy.

Since peanuts can develop the toxic mold when
not properly stored, you should never eat a moldy or
shriveled peanut. In addition, you should be cautious
about—and may want to avoid—eating unroasted peanuts sold in bulk.

IRRADIATION

While some consumers are squeamish about buying produce that carries the stamp of "irradiation," the
process—according to the FDA—reduces or elimi-
nates bacteria, insects, and parasites. It also reduces
spoilage in certain fruits and vegetables and has been
approved by the FDA to prevent sprouting and delay
the ripening process. (Lettuce would wilt and berries

would melt into mush if they were irradiated at levels high enough to kill all *E. coli* bacteria.) For the past eleven years it's been approved for use on vegetables and fruits, but it hasn't caught on in large part because of consumer edginess about safety.

Irradiation does not make food "radioactive," interfere with nutrition, or noticeably change food's taste, texture, or appearance as long as it's properly applied, according to the FDA. In addition to reducing *E. coli* 0157:H7, it controls *Salmonella* and *Campylobacter* as well.

Still, retail stores have been slow to carry irradiated produce because of the belief that customers won't accept the practice, since they fear anything that has to do with radiation. Also, irradiated products have cost slightly more than untreated vegetables and fruits because of the extra step, but these costs should be offset by improved shelf life.

According to the FDA, irradiating food is similar to sending luggage through an airport scanner. The amount of energy isn't strong enough to add any radioactive material to the food. American astronauts have eaten irradiated food since 1972.

WHAT YOU CAN DO

While growers and grocers have their own rules to follow, there are plenty of things you can do to make sure your produce is as nontoxic as possible.

Juices and Cider

Choose only pasteurized juices and cider (more than 98 percent of all fruit and vegetable juices are already pasteurized). Although many top brands don't mention this on the labels of their refrigerated and shelved brands of juice, most—including Juicy Juice, Seneca, Snapple, Veryfine, and Season's Best—are pasteurized.

However, fresh-pressed juices and ciders you buy at a health food store, farm stand, or green market may not be pasteurized. In grocery stores, you may find unpasteurized juice in the refrigerated sections or on ice in the fresh fruits and vegetables section. You can buy these, but once you get home you will have to boil them and then refrigerate.

People in high-risk groups in particular should drink only pasteurized juices. Children on field trips to apple cider mills or farm markets should not be allowed to drink unpasteurized cider.

Vegetables and Fruits

The best way to avoid pesticide contamination is to buy and eat only organically grown produce. (Look for a "certified organic" symbol on the label.) A few states actually have laws legally defining this term. You can also find organic food by mail order; it is usually shipped directly from field to your house.

If you buy vegetables from your store's salad bar, don't select any produce that is brown, dried out, or slimy. These conditions suggest that the items have been held at improper temperatures.

If you want to find out whether your market's fruit and vegetables have been sprayed with pesticides after harvest, you could try asking the market to check the crates, although this information is not always printed there. If your market can't provide this information, shop at one that specializes in organic or locally grown produce.

What About Waxes?

You may notice a thin coating of wax on some fruits and vegetables. This is applied to keep the produce fresh longer by sealing in moisture. It is not applied just to make the items look attractive. You'll likely find the following items coated in wax: apples, cucumbers, grapefruit, melons, oranges, peaches, rutabagas, squash, and tomatoes.

These waxes are regulated by the FDA as "food additives" that are "generally recognized as safe" (GRAS). However, some consumers are worried about the health safety of these waxes, and vegetarians are concerned that the waxes may contain animal-based ingredients. Others worry that the waxes may trap pesticides, despite FDA findings to the contrary.

If you want to avoid waxes, you should know that the FDA requires produce packers and grocers to provide information about waxes on fresh fruits and vegetables. This information can appear as a label on the individual product, on the packing carton (if used at the point of sale), or on counter cards or signs. The information will say that the product is either:

- coated with food-grade, animal-based wax, or
- coated with food-grade vegetable, petroleum-, bees-wax-, and/or shellac-based wax or resin.

In addition, the FDA allows a statement saying that "no wax or resin coating" is used on produce that is free from such coatings.

If your produce does have a coating of wax, you can rinse the fruits and vegetables with warm water and (when appropriate) scrub with a brush to remove most of the wax.

Store It Carefully

If you've cut, peeled, or otherwise broken apart fruits or vegetables, store them in the refrigerator at 40°F or below. In order to avoid the growth of bacteria or mold, you'll want to keep your produce cool and dry. If you have bought fruits or vegetables in plastic wrap, be sure to open the bag so air can circulate.

While you can—and should—store most vegetables and fruits in the refrigerator, you should not put bananas or potatoes in the refrigerator. Likewise, fresh tomatoes shouldn't be stored in the refrigerator; it will affect their taste. Instead, store out of direct sunlight on the counter.

Clean It!

There are other steps you can take to cut down your risk of microbe or pesticide contamination.

Before handling food, wash your hands, and then rinse the produce in warm water for 15 to 30 seconds. (Don't use soap or detergents.) If necessary, use a small scrub brush to remove surface dirt—reserve this brush just for produce. Do this even for prewashed, prepackaged lettuce, and for any fruit you'd peel (such as oranges or bananas), because bacteria living on the peel can be pushed into the fruit when it's cut open.

However, scientists say that colonies of harmful microbes can hide beneath the surface of your produce as you wash it. This can mean that washing produce may not be enough to prevent food-borne illness, according to some U.S. scientists. Research presented at a recent international conference indicated that rinsing fruit didn't completely eliminate the harmful bacteria. For example, most people had rinsed their raspberries that caused outbreaks of cyclosporidiosis in 1996 and 1997.

Other research showed that applying a strong disinfectant for 10 minutes on radish sprouts contaminated with *E. coli* did not eliminate colonies of the bacteria below the surface. (About six thousand Japanese got sick in 1996 after eating *E. coli*–contaminated radish sprouts.)

Discard outer leaves of vegetables like cabbage and lettuce; doing this will reduce by about thirty times the amount of pesticide you ingest.

Serve It Safely
Fruit Juices

Never allow anyone in your family to drink unpasteurized juice, including fresh cider from a roadside stand. Fruit that drops from a tree could land on contaminated feces on the ground; when the fruit is scooped up and pressed for cider, the bacteria can then contaminate many gallons.

Organic Vegetable Wash

If you're worried about what's on your fruits and vegetables, try one of the newest inventions: organic fruit and vegetable wash.

Sold at your grocery store (usually in the produce section), this all-natural spray can help remove surface pesticides, chemicals, dirt, and other harmful substances. The spray has no taste or calories and no alcohol, chlorine, or bleach. It's made from naturally derived cleansers (food-grade fruit and coconut extracts and a natural bio-surfactant).

Simply spray on all fruits and vegetables just before preparing and then rinse with water.

For more information, call 888-VEG-WASH or visit the website at http://www.organiclean.com.

If you do buy unpasteurized cider, boil it for 5 minutes before using. This will kill any bacteria that may exist.

Fruits and Vegetables

Serve a variety of produce so that you can minimize the exposure to specific bacteria and pesticides. Despite widespread concerns about pesticide food contamination, Americans should still eat at least five servings of fruit and vegetables a day, according to the American Dietetic Association, since the benefits far outweigh the risks.

WHAT THE GOVERNMENT IS DOING

While the EPA is in charge of registering and approving pesticides and establishing acceptable residue levels, the FDA is responsible for enforcing the regulations. Under the Federal Insecticide, Fungicide, and Rodenticide Act, the EPA requires manufacturers of new pesticides to submit information about which crops the pesticide is designed for, its effectiveness and toxicity, and the nature and level of residues. The EPA then establishes a tolerance for each pesticide that details how much of the pesticide may legally remain on food crops. The EPA sets acceptable pesticide residue tolerances for each crop or food type on which the pesticide will be used. The same pesticide might have a different tolerance for each fruit and vegetable. The EPA estimates tolerances by figuring out how safe the pesticide is and how much of that particular food you're likely to be eating in one year.

Unfortunately, most pesticides now being used were granted tolerances before safety tests were required to determine whether the pesticide causes cancer, birth defects, genetic damage, or reproductive problems.

The National Academy of Science has voiced serious concerns about the levels of pesticides on food— especially for young consumers. Its report, released in 1993, concludes that the government should be doing a better job of controlling pesticide use on produce. The NAS was especially concerned with the effect of pesticides on infants and children. Because youngsters have smaller bodies and a faster metabolism, federal scientists worry that they may be more susceptible to toxic substances.

As a result of the scientists' findings, the EPA, the FDA, and the USDA have announced a coordinated effort to reduce the use of pesticides in America's food supply. The government's new campaign pledges to improve existing methods of pesticide testing, assessing toxicity risk, and data collection on toxic residues on food. The FDA plans to work on a system to monitor the food supply, and the USDA wants to teach farmers how to use safer pest control methods.

9

Make Sure Your
Water's Safe

Up until the last few years, nobody thought too much about the safety of the water that came out of the tap. But a growing number of waterborne outbreaks have changed all that. It seems that just about everyone agrees that the purity of the drinking water in this country is declining, what with waterborne bacteria, parasites, and viruses, many of which were almost unknown a few years ago.

At the same time, more and more Americans are becoming susceptible to waterborne pathogens. In most healthy people, the damage may be limited to a bout of stomach distress that is often mistaken for the flu. However, for cancer patients, those infected with HIV or suffering from AIDS or other chronic illnesses, as well as the very young and the old, tainted drinking water can be deadly.

Indeed, the Environmental Protection Agency and the Centers for Disease Control and Prevention issued a recent report warning that tap water could be life-threatening to the 5 million Americans with impaired immune systems.

According to the CDC, between 900 and 1,000 people every year die and another million get sick from microbes in their drinking water. Other estimates have put deaths as high as 1,200 and estimated illnesses among Americans at more than 7 million, many never reported to doctors.

In the past, the safety of tap water had been a concern mostly in rural areas, where water systems are less well regulated and private wells are prevalent. But today, the EPA has estimated that 30 million Americans may be drinking from public water systems that violate at least one health standard.

SHOULD YOU HAVE
YOUR WATER TESTED?

Odds are, if your water is contaminated you probably don't know it, since many potential dangers can't be seen or smelled.

If You Have a Private Well

If you drink from a private well, you should have your own water tested once a year. It's best not to go to a company that sells water purification systems—it may have a vested interest in the results. Instead, send your water to an independent lab. You can find one by calling your state health department and asking for names of state-certified independent labs that test for common contaminants. Most tests should cost between

$50 and $150, although a simple test for *E. coli* may cost only $10 or $15.

Having your water tested for some of the new microbes may be more difficult. Only a few labs in the United States can check for *Cryptosporidium*; if your lab can, remember that the test is expensive, often inaccurate, and not very meaningful—the parasite could appear in your water the day after you have it tested. It's probably almost impossible to find a lab that tests for *Helicobacter pylori*, since it has been only very recently that scientists have shown it contaminates surface water.

If You Use Public Water

If you drink public water, you can ask your water company to send you the latest copy of its testing report. All public water companies must test for contamination and report the results to state or federal agencies. The report should include measures of bacteria, total dissolved solids, chemicals, nitrates, pesticides, radioactivity, radium, radon, uranium, trihalomethanes and chloroform, metals, minerals (including fluoride), and alkalinity.

You can check to see if the measurements are below the EPA's maximum allowable limits. (These normally will appear beside the levels in the water tested.) If the normal limits don't appear, you can get a list from the EPA by calling 800-426-4791.

If you're still not satisfied, you can always have your water tested by an independent lab. No matter how safe the water coming into your house is, if you have old pipes that may have lead solder, you need to have your

Symptoms of Troubled Water

If you have too much iron in your water, the sign will be obvious: bright red water. Other contaminants may be harder to observe. Here are some clues:

- oily: industrial chemicals
- perfume/chemical taste: industrial chemicals
- gas smell: leaking underground gas tank
- rotten-egg smell: sewage or hydrogen sulfide contamination
- metallic taste: iron or manganese
- salty taste: road salt contamination
- cloudy water: too much organic material or inadequate purification
- blue-green stain in sink: lead, brass, or copper contaminants
- black fixtures or laundry: high manganese level
- black, pitted stainless-steel sink: too much chloride
- chlorine smell: too much chlorine added to water
- foamy water: septic tank discharge polluting water

water tested for lead contamination by an independent lab. The public system's water tests won't have any validity for your own lead levels. (See section on lead below.)

WHAT TO DO IF YOUR TEST IS POSITIVE

If your water test reveals that your water is contaminated with bacteria, pesticides, radiation, iron, or other problems, you'll need to buy a good water filtration system.

There is a wide variety of water filtration systems that you can buy. Some attach to the pipes under your sink and others can filter all the water coming into your home. Or you can get just a small filtered pitcher for drinking water, if that's all you're worried about.

Filtration systems range in complexity from a simple activated charcoal filter to a complicated reverse osmosis; the best choice is a combination filtration system. Bacterial contamination can be controlled by ultraviolet light attachments. It's important to select the type of system that is designed to solve the particular water problem you have.

If you're interested in a filtration system but you'd like some outside verification that the equipment will really do what it claims, you can contact either the National Sanitation Foundation of Ann Arbor, Michigan, or the Water Quality Association in Lisle, Illinois (see Appendix B for addresses).

TREATMENT SYSTEMS

Activated Carbon Filters

These filters are some of the most-often used, and are a very effective way to remove pesticide contamination from your water supply. An activated carbon filter is the best way to remove bad tastes or odors, not to mention a whole variety of chemical contaminants. However, they are not the best way to remove bacterial contamination from your water. Many systems combine this type of filter with a reverse-osmosis one.

You can buy a carbon filter for your countertop, and simply pour drinking water through it. Or you can attach a filter system under your sink to the cold water line. Never attach a carbon filter to the hot water line, since the temperature can damage the carbon filter cartridge. Shower water, however, is not hot enough to damage a carbon filter; this means you can attach a carbon filter to your shower head to screen out toxic chemicals.

When buying a carbon filter, check the phenol and iodine ratings; the higher the iodine number (it should be at least 1,000) the better at removing toxic chemicals, and the lower the phenol number (no more than 15), the better.

Reverse-Osmosis Filters

These filters are a very good way to remove up to 99 percent of a variety of contaminants, including bacteria, organic and inorganic material, and particles. Reverse-osmosis filters have been shown to be very effective with pesticides and lead. They are less effective at removing trihalomethanes and chloroform, which slip through the membrane; this is why RO systems are often combined with activated carbon.

Ultraviolet Treatment

If bacteria are your problem, ultraviolet radiation can eliminate most microbes and prevent their reproduction. However, some parasites and viruses can survive ultraviolet radiation. Your ultraviolet radiation system should have a "prefilter" to screen out particles, which could otherwise cut down on the system's ability to kill bacteria. It should also have an absorption monitor to warn you if it's absorbing too much ultraviolet radiation.

WHAT IF THERE'S AN OUTBREAK?

If your water comes from a public water system, your utility company is obligated to let you know of an outbreak of microbes in your water. If this happens, boiling the water for one minute will kill the germs—or you can buy bottled water until the emergency is over. You should listen to local radio or TV reports to find out how long you must boil your water to be safe.

HARD OR SOFT WATER?

Many folks these days have a water softener to help them cope with hard water—that is, water with high levels of calcium, magnesium, and other minerals.

How do you know what kind of water you have? Suspect hard water if you have to work hard to get a lather, or if there's sticky, gummy stuff on your pipes and bathtub, or hard white deposits in your pots and coffeemaker.

Hard water can be rough on your appliances, clogging pipes and shortening the life span of your dishwasher or washing machine because of mineral deposit buildups. But nutritionists now believe drinking hard water can be good for your health, reducing the risk of heart disease.

You might consider getting a water softener to attach to those pipes that feed into appliances, but bypassing the pipe that goes to your kitchen faucet.

Remember that water softeners don't remove toxic contaminants; they simply remove calcium and magnesium. If you opt for this system you should know it may increase the salt level in your water by up to five times the amount. If you're on a low-sodium diet, you may find that this water will raise your sodium intake.

WHAT ABOUT BOTTLED WATER?

Some people have given up on drinking tap water altogether, and choose to drink bottled water instead. However, there are a dizzying array of types and brands to choose from. In fact, there are just about as many different kinds of bottled water as there are brands of beer.

- *Artesian well water* is water from a confined, underground water source.

Coliform Count

The coliform count is a method of determining the level of fecal coliform bacteria *(E. coli)* in water. These bacteria are common in our lower intestines, but they should not be found in our water.

Commonly, ocean water along public beaches is tested regularly in the summer for coliform bacteria. Contaminated water can prompt the authorities to close beaches, since the bacteria can cause disease.

- *Distilled water* has been vaporized and then condensed back into water.
- *Mineral water* is from an underground source and contains minerals (such as sodium and calcium).
- *Sparkling water* is filtered tap or spring water that has been or is naturally carbonated.
- *Spring water* is from an underground source from which water flows naturally to the surface.

Distillation kills microbes, including *Cryptosporidium*, and makes water especially safe for rinsing contact lenses. But except for distilled water, no one type of water is any more pure or healthier than another. In fact, federal standards for bottled water are only slightly more stringent than for municipal water. On the other hand, many people believe bottled water tastes better than tap water because bottlers use ozone to disinfect their water, not chlorine. Ozone leaves no taste or odor, but it's rarely used in public water systems because it becomes less effective once it hits the air.

If you do choose bottled water, you'll want to make sure the bottler is a member of the Bottled Water Association, a trade group that monitors the quality of the water of its members. Want to know if the company that makes your favorite brand belongs? Call 800-WATER-11.

IS CHLORINE SAFE?

If you have public water gushing out of your faucet, odds are it's treated with chlorine, which probably affects its taste and smell, depending on the level of microbes in your water supply. Most experts agree that small amounts of chlorine in your drinking water probably won't hurt you.

What's less clear is what happens when that chlorine mixes with the residue from decaying leaves and other organic matter in public systems that utilize reservoirs and other open bodies of water. In one 1992 study, researchers found that people who regularly drank tap water containing high levels of chlorine by-products had a higher chance of developing bladder and rectal cancers than those who drank unchlorinated water.

More recent studies have suggested that pregnant women who drink water tainted with these by-products have a higher risk of miscarriages. To be safe, if you're pregnant you might want to consider drinking only bottled water until the baby is born.

PESTICIDES IN WATER

Some studies have found that at certain times of the year in certain parts of the country—especially in the Midwest—tap water in many cities carries testable levels of pesticides, including weed-killers, that are above the EPA safety levels. This is also a considerable problem in rural areas, where well water may be contaminated by runoff from fields.

Young children and babies are at particular risk because of their developmental stage. If you live in a farming region, you may want to think about using bottled water—especially for pregnant and nursing women, babies, and young children—at least from May through August.

LEAD IN WATER

Lead in water is not a problem of the past; lead is still leaching into drinking water from pipes, faucets, and well pumps. In fact, the EPA estimates that about 15 percent of U.S. families have too much lead in their water, which can cause developmental problems and learning disabilities in children under age six.

If you live in a home built before 1930, you're at the very highest risk, since pipes from that time and before were made of lead. However, any house built before 1988 could have some lead in the water because of lead solder in the pipes. The main problems are corroded lead plumbing, lead solder on copper plumbing, and brass faucets. However, as late as 1988 some parts of the country (such as Chicago and Washington, D.C.) still built houses using lead service connections. If you have a lead service connection at your house, let the water run for between two and five minutes (or until the temperature changes) to flush your service connectors.

The EPA rules state that if lead exceeds 15 parts per billion in more than 10 percent of the public water taps sampled, then the system must begin a series of corrosion control treatments. (For bottled water, the FDA requires that lead not be present at a rate about 5 ppb, the lowest concentration that water analysis can reliably measure. Bottled water with more lead than this is removed from the market.)

If you suspect you do have a problem, turn the water on first thing in the morning and let it run for a minute or two before you use it. This way, you're flushing out the water that's been sitting overnight in the pipes, accumulating lead. Use cold water for drinking and cooking, running it 30 seconds before each use. When you're finished doing the dishes in the evening, fill up a bottle of water and leave it uncovered overnight; this is the purest water you'll have. You can use it the next morning for making coffee or reconstituting juice.

Likewise, if lead is a problem at your house, you should never use hot water from the tap when you're making baby formula, since hot water will have higher lead concentrations.

Ask your state health agency about testing your drinking water for lead.

10

Those at Special Risk

As we've seen so far, the problem of microorganisms in food and water is a growing concern across the nation. But while most cases of food poisoning in healthy young adults aren't serious, they are a far different matter in high-risk individuals.

These high-risk people include pregnant women, nursing mothers, young children and infants, the elderly, patients with certain chronic health conditions (such as liver disease, diabetes, and cancer), and those with impaired immune systems—AIDS patients, organ transplant patients, and people on long-term steroid therapy or chemotherapy. This chapter will discuss the special issues of food-borne illness for those at special risk.

SAFE EATING HABITS
FOR AT-RISK PEOPLE

- Never eat raw meat, poultry, or seafood. Especially dangerous are raw oysters and raw clams.
- Don't eat raw or undercooked eggs, or any dishes that contain them. These include Caesar salads, mousse, custards, homemade ice cream containing raw eggs, and homemade mayonnaise.
- Avoid soft cheeses, such as feta, Brie, Camembert, blue, or Mexican-style soft white cheese (like queso blanco or queso fresco); but you can eat hard cheese, processed slices, cottage cheese, and yogurt.
- Never eat hamburgers that are pink inside.
- Don't eat at deli counters.

SAFE COOKING HABITS
FOR AT-RISK PEOPLE

- Make sure stuffing inside poultry has been heated to at least 165°F.
- Thoroughly reheat lunch meats and hot dogs.
- Never leave food out at room temperature for more than two hours.
- Keep cold food cold and hot food hot.

TYPES OF FOOD-BORNE ILLNESS

Certain types of food-borne illness are of particular concern to high-risk consumers: salmonellosis, campylobacteriosis, cryptosporidiosis, and listeriosis.

Salmonellosis

Infection with *Salmonella* is the most common cause of food-borne illness, and while it can affect anyone, it occurs almost a hundred times more often in people with AIDS than in other people. When salmonellosis does strike an AIDS patient, it is especially hard to treat and may be more likely to lead to serious complications.

Campylobacteriosis

Infection with *Campylobacter*, often a result of the improper handling or cooking of poultry, can be serious in persons with impaired immunity. *Campylobacter* can also be found in a wide variety of other foods. When it strikes persons with impaired immunity, it is usually severe and often fatal.

Cryptosporidiosis

Cryptosporidium exists in many forms, and experts aren't certain exactly how it finds its way into the nation's water supplies. When it does, it can make lots of people sick—but it's hardest on the at-risk individual.

Large-scale purification systems for city water supplies (including elaborate filtration devices) haven't solved the problem, and routine chlorination won't eliminate cryptosporidiosis.

Many at-risk people drink bottled water, but not all bottled water brands provide a safe alternative to boiling. Remember that unless it's distilled or pasteurized, bottled water may not be any safer than tap water. Current standards for bottled water don't guarantee that the water is free of contamination from *Cryptosporidium*.

If an outbreak of *Cryptosporidium* has been announced for your area, high-risk patients should listen carefully to all advisories issued by the state health department. Boiling water for at least one minute at a rolling boil will kill *Cryptosporidium*. If you get your water from a properly drilled and maintained well, the water is usually protected from surface contamination and is not likely to contain the cysts.

There is indication that some water filters may help prevent, or lessen the risk of, cryptosporidiosis. During the outbreak in Milwaukee in 1993, one study found that people who used water filters with a pore size less than 2 microns had less diarrhea than those who used filters with larger pore sizes.

If you want to be sure that your filtration unit can remove *Crypto*, it should carry one of the following four messages:

- "reverse osmosis"
- "absolute pore size of 1 micron or smaller"
- "tested and certified by NSF Standard 53 for cyst removal"
- "tested and certified by NSF Standard 53 for cyst reduction"

If you do use a home filter, follow the manufacturer's instructions, which will give you details on filter maintenance. Filters should be certified by the National Sanitation Foundation, or an equivalent testing agency.

For more information about filters for *Cryptosporidium*, call the CDC AIDS Hotline at 800-342-2437.

Listeriosis

One of the most dangerous food-borne illnesses a pregnant woman can contract is caused by *Listeria monocytogenes* bacteria. These bacteria can cause conditions that lead to miscarriage or illness in newborns. They have been found in unpasteurized milk, imported soft cheeses and other deli-type cheeses, hot dogs, lunch meats, spreads, and other processed meats.

Listeriosis strikes about 1,850 Americans each year and causes 460 deaths as a result of blood poisoning, meningitis, flulike illnesses, complications of pregnancy, and stillbirths. The amount of microbes necessary to cause illness is not known, but experts think it varies with the strain of *Listeria* and the vulnerability of the patient. However, experts believe that in at-risk individuals, less than 1,000 organisms may cause disease.

In high-risk patients, *Listeria* meningitis kills as many as 70 percent of its victims. Blood poisoning, another complication of listeriosis, kills 50 percent of all who develop it and 80 percent of infected infants.

One recent study found that 20 percent of hot dogs tested contained the bacterium *L. monocytogenes*. Testing for *Listeria* usually involves sampling foods and monitoring food processing plants; such testing can pinpoint locations that require extra attention. New, rapid tests can confirm the presence of *Listeria* within twenty-four hours.

To control *Listeria*, you should be sure to promptly refrigerate all food that needs cold storage. Don't buy or use any food that has passed its "use by" date. Throw out any sealed, unopened lunch meats or spreads that have been sitting in the refrigerator for more than two weeks after you bought them. Use or discard any open packages in three to four days.

PREGNANT WOMEN

Any illness a pregnant woman contracts can affect her unborn child, whose immune system is too immature to fight back. In addition to the extra risks for the infections listed above, there are some unique problems pregnant women face in connection with water.

According to a recent study, pregnant women in their first trimester who drink five or more glasses of cold tap water a day can be at a higher risk for miscarriage if their water supply has a contaminant called trihalomethane. This contaminant forms when chlorine reacts with acids from plants, and it's found in chlorinated water in most municipal water systems across the country. It is usually a problem in public water systems that get their water from large lakes or reservoirs where plant matter collects.

The miscarriage risk was calculated at 15.7 percent, compared to a risk of 9.5 percent in the general population. As a result, pregnant women were advised that if they drank that much tap water, they might want to boil the water first and keep it in the refrigerator. Carbon-filtered water can be left in the refrigerator for several hours before drinking.

IMPAIRED IMMUNITY

Of all high-risk individuals, AIDS patients are among the most vulnerable to food-borne infections. As the virus damages the immune system, the patient becomes vulnerable to infection by food-borne bacteria and other microbes, as well as parasites. Three types of bacteria are of particular concern for persons with AIDS: *Salmonella*, *Campylobacter*, and *Listeria*.

Salmonellosis can affect anyone, but it's found almost a hundred times more often in people with AIDS; when it does occur, it can be especially difficult to treat and is more likely to lead to serious complications.

Illnesses caused by *Campylobacter* infection occur about thirty-five times more often in AIDS patients. The infection often stems from poor handling or cooking of poultry. Contaminated drinking water is another source of this infection.

Listeria infections are also much more common in people with AIDS, and are profoundly severe and usually fatal in this high-risk population. Because the risk from *Listeria* in this group is so high, some patients choose to avoid all foods that may contain the bacteria, including deli meats and cheeses and hot dogs.

Other food-borne illnesses that can affect AIDS patients include hepatitis A, giardiasis, and shellfish poisoning. The actual extent to which people who are infected with the human immunodeficiency virus (HIV) are at higher risk is not known, but experts believe that any additional infection can hasten the progression from HIV infection to autoimmune deficiency syndrome (AIDS).

People with AIDS need to take special precautions when traveling abroad. You should:

- boil all water
- drink only canned or carbonated beverages, and use only ice made from boiled water
- avoid uncooked vegetables and salads
- peel all fruit
- cook all food thoroughly and eat while it's still hot

CHILDREN

The Centers for Disease Control and Prevention estimates that half of all infections with the deadly *E. coli* bacteria strike children under age fifteen. In general, the younger the child, the higher the risk of serious food-borne illness and complications because of an undeveloped immune system.

Of course, all of the food safety precautions outlined in Chapters 2 and 3 hold true for children as well. But there are also some special precautions.

Baby Food
Homemade Baby Food

Making your baby's food can be a healthy choice, but you also need to be extremely careful not to contaminate that food. Make sure all your equipment (including grinders, blenders, counters, can openers, and so on) is clean; old food bits can harbor bacteria that could cause disease. Thoroughly rinse equipment with very hot water.

When you puree or grind up food for baby, bacteria are more likely to grow in the food because of the increased surface area. Therefore, limit the length of time baby food is stored in the freezer or refrigerator. Don't refreeze pureed food, because it could spoil.

Handling Baby Food and Formula Safely

Remember never to give baby leftovers from a previous bottle feeding, since harmful bacteria from your baby's mouth could have gotten into the formula, where it will grow even after refrigeration and reheating. That's also why you don't want to feed baby straight from a jar of baby food; baby saliva can mix with the food. Maybe you have eaten right from a can more than once, but remember that an infant's immune system is not as strong as yours; even a small dose of harmful bacteria can make a very young infant extremely sick.

Storing Baby Food

It's a good idea to observe all "use by" dates stamped on unopened cans of formula or unopened jars. You can store evaporated milk for up to a year. Make sure the safety button on the baby food jar is still down before opening; if the jar lid doesn't "pop" when you open it, it wasn't sealed safely. Throw the food out.

Microwaving Baby Food

Don't heat liquids in disposable bottles in the microwave; heat in hot tap water instead. Don't heat meats, meat sticks, eggs, or jars of food intended for baby in the microwave, either. Hot spots could burn a young child.

Transfer baby food from the jar into a heat dish; for 4 ounces of food, microwave on high 15 seconds, stir, and then let it stand for at least 30 seconds. Always stir and then test the temperature of the food.

Day Care and Safety from Infection

Most American children are in day care, and experts say that by the year 1999, eight out of ten youngsters will spend at least some time there. While it may be a necessity, day care can pose some extra risks for youngsters. Because young children have immature immune systems, they tend to become infected with any virus or bacterium that happens to be in their vicinity.

A day care situation is a prime breeding ground for infection because of the large numbers of children in close quarters, the shared use of toys and blankets, and diapering and food activities.

For this reason, when you're looking for a day care center, see if the workers have taken any special training in first aid and food handling. The American Red Cross, the American Academy of Pediatrics, and

Safe Storage for Baby Food

Food	Refrigerator	Freezer
Strained fruits/ vegetables	2–3 days	6–8 months
Strained meats/ eggs	1 day	1–2 months
Meat/vegetable combo	1–2 days	1–2 months
Homemade baby foods	1–2 days	3–4 months
Expressed breast milk	5 days	3–4 months
Formula	2 days	Not recommended
Whole milk	5 days	3 months

the National Academy of Science have developed an accredited child care course to train child care workers in first aid, food handling, and preventing infectious diseases. (For more information, contact your local Red Cross.) In some situations, scholarships can be arranged for qualified applicants.

"Bugs" in Day Care

There are several types of microbes that are particularly problematic in day care situations. The most common is *Shigella*, the bacteria that causes diarrhea. *Shigella* can be transmitted by infected people to food or water, and may cause up to 20,000 reported cases of food poisoning a year, mostly in children under age four. Other microbes include *Giardia, E. coli,* and those causing hepatitis A and common viral infections.

Judging Your Child's Day Care

In well-run centers, there should be a set of important health rules that are standard operating procedure, according to the American Red Cross and government agencies:

- Good refrigeration and reheating facilities should be available for food and beverages.
- Toilet areas (and diaper changing areas) should be clean and away from food preparation areas.
- Used diapers and wipes should be stored in closed containers and removed daily.
- Items that go into children's mouths should be sanitized often.
- Children should never share tissues or washcloths;

their personal belongings should be labeled and separated.

- There should be ample space for ventilation between cribs, beds, cots, and nap rugs; children should sleep in positions alternating heads and feet.
- Centers should require all up-to-date vaccinations, and have a well-defined policy on illness exclusion.
- Centers should serve food sent from home only if it is properly covered and refrigerated and looks safe and wholesome.
- Teachers and children should wash their hands before eating and after toileting.
- Children should not share food or utensils.

What You Can Do

There are also some things you can do to help protect your child. Put your baby's formula in a bottle with her name on it, cap and refrigerate, and place in the center's refrigerator as soon as you get there. Make sure any perishable snacks are refrigerated at the center. Instruct your child on the importance of handwashing after toileting and before eating.

SENIORS

As we mature, our bodies change and the immune system becomes less effective, less able to ward off infections. And once ill, older people take longer to recover from an illness. Some of the changes that seniors experience affect the way the body can fight bacteria—for example, the secretion of stomach acid drops,

Manual for Day Care Centers

To improve overall standards for day care centers and child care professionals, the American Public Health Association and the American Academy of Pediatrics recently issued a comprehensive publication, "National Health and Safety Performance Standards: Guidelines for Out-of-Home Child Care Programs." It covers family day care, group day care, and child care centers and is available from Publication Sales, APHA, 1015 Fifteenth Street NW, Washington DC 20005.

inhibiting the ability to fight ingested bacteria. In addition, the senses of taste and smell may not be keen enough to alert an older person that the food or beverage is spoiled or sour.

By following the safe food handling practices as outlined in Chapters 2 and 3, older people can protect themselves against possibly serious food-borne illness.

11

Types of Food Poisoning

Every day across this country, people prepare, cook, or store food incorrectly, leaving themselves vulnerable for the development of food poisoning. Food can be affected by a variety of contaminants, including bacteria, viruses, and parasites, all of which cause food-borne illness. What kinds of poisoning are we talking about, and how can you tell if you are suffering from food poisoning?

I. BACTERIAL FOOD POISONING

Bacteria can be found in the air, the water, food, and everything we touch. Since few of these are harmful, humans are seldom bothered by them. When harmful bacteria do enter the body, most of the time our immune system kills the invading microbes.

Bacteria come in a variety of shapes, colors, and sizes, and have many ways of living. Some bacteria feed on other organisms, some make their own food (as plants do), and some do both. Some need air to survive and others exist without air. Some move by themselves, and others can't move at all.

Not all bacteria are harmful; most are helpful, such as those that break down dead plant and animal matter in the soil. Bacteria are also used in making cheese out of milk, and leather out of animal hide. Grazing animals use bacteria in their stomachs to digest grass.

Bacteria are of incredible importance because of their extreme flexibility, their capacity for rapid growth and reproduction, and their ancient age—the oldest known fossils are those of bacteria-like organisms that lived nearly 3.5 billion years ago.

Campylobacter Jejuni

Campylobacter was first recognized in the 1970s as a cause of campylobacteriosis, the so-called traveler's diarrhea. Linked to raw and undercooked poultry, unpasteurized milk, and untreated water, this common food-borne illness causes an estimated 4 million infections and 1,000 deaths every year.

While the illness can be uncomfortable and even disabling, deaths occur primarily among those with impaired immune systems, the very young, and the very old. In one of the best-known outbreaks during the 1980s, more than 3,000 residents in Bennington, Vermont, became ill with diarrhea when their town's water supply was contaminated with the rod-shaped bacterium. The disease may also spread throughout child care centers.

Food sources The most common source of infection is contaminated poultry (one-third to one-half of all raw chicken on the market is contaminated). Consumers get sick when they eat undercooked chicken, or when the organisms are transferred from the raw meat or raw meat drippings to the mouth. *Campylobacter* can also survive in undercooked lamb, beef, or pork, in water, and in raw milk.

Onset Symptoms begin from two to ten days after eating tainted food, and may last up to ten days.

Symptoms Fever, headache, and muscle pain followed by sometimes-bloody diarrhea, abdominal pain and nausea, and fatigue and body aches.

Diagnosis The infection is diagnosed by culturing a stool sample.

Treatment Unless antibiotics are taken at the very beginning of the illness they won't affect symptoms, although they will shorten the infectious period. Without treatment, stool is infectious for several weeks, but three days of antibiotics will eliminate the bacteria. For mild cases, rest and fluids should be sufficient. Young children are usually given antibiotics (usually erythromycin) to reduce the risk of passing the infection on to other children.

Complications Occasionally infection may provoke urinary tract infections, meningitis, reactive arthritis, or a paralyzing neurologic illness called Guillain-Barré syndrome.

Prognosis The infection can be fatal. The Centers for Disease Control and Prevention recorded two deaths from outbreaks over a nine-year period.

Prevention Don't drink unpasteurized milk or untreated water from mountain streams or lakes. Use caution when handling and preparing poultry.

Bacillus Cereus

Bacillus cereus bacteria multiply in raw foods at room temperature, producing heat-resistant toxins most often found in steamed or refried rice. While *B. cereus* poisoning is less common in the United States than elsewhere, it's likely that episodes are underreported because symptoms are so similar to other types of food poisoning.

Food sources Cereals (especially rice), vegetables, and pasta.

Symptoms These bacteria produce two distinct types of food poisoning. The first type features a short incubation period after eating tainted food (usually less than six hours) and causes cramps and vomiting, and occasionally a short bout of diarrhea. Almost 80 percent of patients with these symptoms who test positive for *B. cereus* poisoning have eaten steamed or refried rice at Chinese restaurants. The second type appears within eight to twenty-four hours after ingestion of tainted food and causes abdominal cramps and diarrhea with very little vomiting.

Treatment There is no specific therapy beyond treating symptoms.

Complications None.

Prognosis Illness is usually mild and self-limiting.

Prevention Keep preparation surfaces clean, and don't allow leftovers to remain in the open air for long. Heat leftovers quickly, and eat them right away.

Clostridium Botulinum

The deadliest known type of food poisoning is botulism, caused by the *Clostridium botulinum* toxin, the most poisonous substance in the world—six million times more toxic than rattlesnake venom. In fact, the fearsome reputation of botulism is well deserved, since two-thirds of botulism victims die. Those who survive face a long recovery period.

The bacteria's resistance to heat makes the spores an important cause of poisoning from improperly cooked or canned foods. While still fairly uncommon, botulism occurs more often in the United States than anywhere else in the world due to the popularity here of home canning; there are about twenty cases of food-borne botulism in the United States annually.

Botulism occurs when sealed foods aren't processed at high enough temperatures to kill the toxic spores, which are harmless until they are deprived of oxygen (e.g., inside a sealed can or jar). Botulism from commercially canned food is rare because of strict health standards enforced by the FDA. Most instances of botulism occur during errors in home canning. The tightly fitted lids of home-canned food provide the anaerobic environment necessary for the growth of botulism toxins, but the spores won't grow if the food is very acidic, sweet, or salty, as in canned fruit juice, jams and jellies, sauerkraut, tomatoes, and heavily salted hams.

Food sources Typically, home-canned green beans, beets, peppers, corn, and meat. While the spores can survive boiling and freezing, the ideal temperature for their growth is between 78°F and 96°F. In addition, the bacteria are commonly found in soil, on plants, and in the intestinal tracts of animals and fish, where the spores can survive for years.

Onset Symptoms may occur as soon as three hours or as late as fourteen days after eating tainted food, but usually appear between eighteen and thirty-six hours after ingestion.

Symptoms Botulism affects the nervous system and only occasionally causes vomiting or diarrhea; primary symptoms are weakness, blurred vision, headache, difficulty swallowing, slurred speech, drooping eyelids, dilated pupils, and paralysis progressing to the respiratory muscles. Symptoms generally last between three and six days; death occurs in about 70 percent of untreated cases, usually due to suffocation.

Treatment Call your local health department immediately in suspected cases of botulism. Induce vomiting immediately upon onset of symptoms; since vomiting may not completely remove the toxin, botulism may still develop. Therefore, prompt administration of the antitoxin lowers the risk of death to 25 percent. The Centers for Disease Control and Prevention in Atlanta handles the antitoxin and makes the decision to treat.

Prognosis The earlier the onset of symptoms, the more severe the reaction. The antitoxin won't reverse paralysis that has already begun, so treatment within twenty-four hours of the onset of symptoms may shorten the course of the poisoning and may prevent total paralysis.

Prevention Proper canning should prevent most cases of botulism.

Botulism (Infant): Clostridium Botulinum

Another type of fatal botulism affects infants who have eaten honey contaminated with *C. botulinum*. For some reason, some infants under age one are highly susceptible to the spores. Research suggests that mother's milk may provide some immunological protection against infant botulism.

Symptoms Constipation, facial muscle flaccidity, sucking problems, irritability, and lethargy.

Prognosis Unfortunately, infant botulism symptoms may go unrecognized by parents until the poisoning has reached a critical stage.

Prevention Never feed children under age one honey, and keep rooms dust free.

Clostridium Perfringens

This type of bacteria, a close cousin of *C. botulinum*, can produce a dangerous toxin that multiplies quickly in reheated foods, which is why it's known as the "cafeteria germ." It's often found in food that is served in large amounts, such as in hospitals and school cafeterias, and in food left in inadequately heated steam tables or at room temperature. Once ingested, the bacteria produce a toxin in the digestive tract about six hours later. However, to cause illness, a large amount of the bacteria must be ingested.

This type of food poisoning is very common in the United States, with an estimated ten thousand cases occurring each year, according to the CDC. Outbreaks have often been traced to restaurants, caterers, and cafeterias that don't have adequate refrigeration facilities. Most cases go unreported.

Food sources Undercooked beef, meat pies, stews, burritos, tacos, enchiladas, and reheated meats or gravies made from beef, turkey, or chicken.

Onset Within eight to twenty-four hours after eating.

Symptoms Severe colic or cramps and abdominal gas pains followed by a twenty-four-hour bout of watery diarrhea. There may be nausea but usually not vomiting or fever.

Diagnosis A test can detect the presence of the bacterium. The bacteria will also grow on a culture plate in a lab from either the food or a stool sample.

Treatment While there is no antitoxin available, some doctors recommend treatment with penicillin. Drink small sips of clear fluids or electrolytes to replace what is lost. If you are dehydrated, seek medical help.

Prognosis While usually a mild illness, *C. perfringens* poisoning can be dangerous to infants and the elderly, who may become dehydrated. You can get this illness more than once, but patients are not infectious.

Prevention The bacteria produce spores, which are a dormant form of bacteria that isn't killed by cooking. However, the spores can't develop into new bacteria at temperatures below 40°F or above 140°F. Therefore, keep hot food hot and cold foods cold and don't keep reheating and reusing leftovers for several meals.

E. Coli 0157:H7

The most deadly of the hundreds of strains of *Escherichia coli*, this type has emerged during the past ten years as a cause of food-borne illness leading to kidney failure and death. It's known popularly as the "hamburger disease" because of its links with undercooked fast-food burgers.

Although most strains of *E. coli* are harmless and live in the intestines of both humans and animals, the 0157:H7 strain produces a powerful toxin that can cause severe illness. An estimated 10,000 to 20,000 cases of infection occur in the United States each year. Most illness has been associated with eating undercooked, contaminated ground beef. The number of these cases appears to be increasing, as has the frequency of complications. Outbreaks occurred in fast-food chain hamburgers in 1993, and in unpasteurized apple cider in 1991. Infection is especially common in day care centers and among toddlers who are not yet toilet trained. Patients are infectious for about six days while bacteria are being excreted in the stool. There is no solid evidence, but it appears that victims can get this infection more than once. About thirty-eight states now ask doctors to report outbreaks of the disease, but none regularly test for other strains of *E. coli* that produce the toxin.

Food sources Outbreaks have been traced to many different types of food; the bacteria can survive in dry fermented meat and salami despite production standards that meet federal and industry food processing requirements. *E. coli* 0157:H7 has been found in un-pasteurized milk, cider, and apple juice; lettuce; and untreated water.

Symptoms Severe cramps and watery or bloody diarrhea lasting for several days. Other symptoms include nausea and vomiting appearing within hours to a week after eating, but not usually any fever. Most people recover quickly and completely, but the complications are what make this a serious disease.

Diagnosis Identification of the bacterium in stool. Most labs that culture stool don't test for *E. coli* 0157:H7, so it's important to request that the stool be tested for this organism. Everyone with sudden bloody diarrhea should have the stool checked for this bacterium.

Treatment Most patients recover within ten days without specific treatment. There is no evidence that antibiotics help, and some evidence to suggest they may trigger kidney problems. Antidiarrhea medicine should also be avoided. HUS (see below) is a life-threatening condition that is treated in a hospital intensive care unit, with blood transfusions and kidney dialysis.

Complications In certain people (the very young or old), the bacteria may cause hemolytic uremia syndrome (HUS), a condition in which the red blood cells are destroyed and the kidneys fail. Between 2 and 7 percent of infections lead to this complication. In the United States, HUS is the main cause of kidney failure in children. There is no cure. Adults may develop an extremely serious bleeding disorder called thrombotic thrombocytopenic purpura in which blood stops clotting, small red spots and large bruises appear all over the body, and blood oozes from the mouth.

Prognosis Patients with only a mild *E. coli* 0157:H7 infection usually recover completely. Of those who develop HUS, one-third have abnormal kidney function years later and a few need long-term dialysis. Another 8 percent suffer with other complications, such as high blood pressure, seizures, blindness, and paralysis, for the rest of their lives. Even with intensive care, the death rate from HUS is between 3 and 5 percent. In addition, the outlook is not promising for adults who develop thrombotic thrombocytopenic purpura.

Helicobacter Pylori

This bacterium, which causes most stomach ulcers and almost all duodenal ulcers, is believed to exist in groundwater throughout the United States. In 1983, the bacterium was found in the stomach tissue of ulcer patients. While half the world's populations are believed to be infected (including an estimated 40 million Americans), *Helicobacter pylori* causes ulcers in only 10 to 20 percent of its hosts. Still, one out of every ten Americans has an ulcer, and *H. pylori* is implicated in 90 percent of those cases.

Food source Groundwater.

Symptoms Nausea and stomach pain, vomiting and fever lasting between three and fourteen days. Virtually everyone with the bacteria has chronic gastritis (a mild inflammation of the stomach lining), which may last for decades. Some people with the infection don't have ulcers but do have nausea, gas, bloating, and burning stomach pain.

Diagnosis Blood tests can determine the presence of antibodies to the bacteria, which indicate whether you have ever had the infection but not whether it's active. A biopsy can reveal *H. pylori*. Breath tests are currently being studied and may be available in the near future.

Treatment About 90 percent of *H. pylori* infections can be cured with a combination of antiulcer medication (Pepto-Bismol) and specific antibiotics (metronidazole, and either tetracycline or amoxicillin). However, the treatment is not easy; it involves taking twelve to sixteen pills for two weeks and carries the risk of some side effects, such as fatigue and dizziness. Because the treatment may not be completely successful, follow-up testing at least four weeks after completing treatment may be needed to make sure the bacteria are no longer present. If tests reveal no bacteria, the patient is not likely to be reinfected ever again. Persistent infection may require a different medication for a longer period of time.

Complications The organism has also been found in a disproportionately large number of patients with certain kinds of stomach cancer. Some scientists suggest the infection may triple the risk of this rare cancer. While there appears to be a relationship between the bacteria and stomach cancer, these cancers are becoming less common in the United States and therapy for *H. pylori* has not been recommended as a preventive measure.

Prevention Chlorine in public drinking water kills the bacteria, but shallow wells may be contaminated by surface water tainted with them (deeper wells are less likely to have the bacteria). Normal water-testing procedures can't identify the presence of *H. pylori*, and there is no test at present that you can use on your well. However, private labs can test water for microscopic particulates, which will determine if the well water has been contaminated with surface water, and thus by bacteria. You can install an ultraviolet disinfection system to treat contaminated water. Charcoal-based tap filters may not be a good choice, because bacteria can grow on the charcoal.

Listeria Monocytogenes

Listeriosis is one of the most dangerous food-borne illnesses a pregnant woman can contract, causing conditions that can lead to miscarriage or to illness in the newborn baby. The government estimates that there are about 1,600 cases of listeriosis each year, and 415 deaths. Some studies have suggested that as many as 10 percent of all Americans carry the bacteria in their intestines.

While pregnant women are most at risk, others at high risk include people with a compromised immune system, cancer patients (especially leukemia patients), the elderly, and people with diabetes, cirrhosis of the liver, asthma, or ulcerative colitis.

There have been outbreaks traced to Mexican-style cheese in California that led to numerous stillbirths, as well as a cluster of cases in Philadelphia.

Food sources Unpasteurized milk, imported soft cheese, hot dogs, lunch meats and spreads, raw vegetables, fermented raw-meat sausage, raw and cooked poultry, raw meats, and raw or smoked fish. One recent study found that 20 percent of hot dogs tested contained the bacterium. When *Listeria* is found in processed products, the contamination probably occurred after processing (rather than due to poor heating or pasteurizing).

Onset Illness occurs within three weeks after consuming the tainted product.

Symptoms Most healthy people probably don't show any symptoms. Flulike symptoms, including a persistent fever, appear first. Nausea, vomiting, and diarrhea may precede more serious forms of listeriosis, or may be the only symptoms. In high-risk individuals, the infection may spread to the nervous system, causing a type of meningitis that includes intense headache, fever, stiff neck, confusion, loss of balance, or convulsions. *Listeria* meningitis carries a fatality rate that may reach 70 percent.

Diagnosis Listeriosis can be diagnosed from a blood test, cerebrospinal fluid, or stool. There is no routine screening test for susceptibility during pregnancy.

Treatment Antibiotics are most helpful in pregnant women to prevent disease in the fetus. Babies with listeriosis receive the same antibiotics as adults, although a combination of antibiotics may be used until diagnosis is certain. Even with prompt treatment, some infections result in death, especially in those with other serious medical problems.

Complications Internal abscesses, meningitis, blood poisoning. In pregnant women, the infection can lead to stillbirth or miscarriage.

Prognosis Listeriosis can be very serious and can be fatal.

Prevention Avoid high-risk foods if you are pregnant or a patient with an impaired immune system. Practice good food preparation practices and wash all vegetables and salads well.

Plesiomonas Shigelloides

This bacterium is found in water, freshwater fish, and shellfish; it causes a type of gastroenteritis among people in tropical or subtropical regions. Because most infections are mild, people don't seek medical treatment. It is not commonly reported in the United States, but this may be because cases are included in a group of diarrhea diseases of unknown origin that respond to broad-spectrum antibiotics. Many cases reported in the United States involve people with preexisting health problems or very young patients.

Food source Most cases appear to be related to tainted water that is consumed or used to rinse vegetables eaten raw.

Onset Usually within a day or two after eating or drinking tainted food.

Symptoms Fever, chills, abdominal pain, nausea, watery diarrhea, or vomiting. In severe cases, diarrhea may be foamy, greenish-yellow, or tinged with blood. While the diarrhea is mild in most people, in infants and young children it may be accompanied by high fever and chills; blood poisoning and death have occurred among those who have faulty immune systems or who are seriously ill with cancer or blood disorders.

Treatment Most people recover on their own.

Salmonella

Typically associated with a very wide range of foods, salmonellosis is caused by one of the more than 2,300 strains (*Salmonella enteritidis* and *S. typhimurium* are the most common) that multiply rapidly at room temperature. It's responsible for more than 2 million infections and between 500 and 2,000 deaths each year. Especially worrisome is an outbreak of a new drug-resistant strain (*Salmonella typhimurium* DT 104).

Food sources Raw or undercooked poultry and eggs, raw meats, fish, nonpasteurized milk, and any foods made from them. Large outbreaks have occurred in egg-containing foods in California in 1995, in mass-distributed ice cream in 1994, and in mass-distributed cantaloupes in 1989.

Onset From twelve hours to eight days after eating contaminated food.

Symptoms Severe headache, nausea, fever, stomach cramps, diarrhea, vomiting, and sometimes a rash. Symptoms usually last two to seven days. The infection can be fatal in infants and the elderly.

Treatment There's not much you can do for salmonellosis except treat symptoms: eat a bland diet (liquids and soft solids) and drink plenty of fluids to offset dehydration. Antibiotic treatment (chloramphenicol, ampicillin, or a tetracycline) should be administered only in cases of severe infection, or to people at high risk for complications.

Complications Meningitis, blood poisoning, bone/joint infections.

Prognosis Infection may be mild to severe, and can be fatal (especially in very young or very old patients, or people with impaired immune systems).

Prevention Prepare and cook chicken, eggs, and other poultry and meats correctly; don't leave food out in room temperature.

Shigella

Shigellosis is caused by four different species of bacteria. *Shigella* is common in developing countries where lack of sewage treatment is linked to contaminated food and water. It is less common in the United States, but still causes about 300,000 cases each year. The disease is very common among AIDS patients, and it's most serious among them, and the very young and old. A person gets sick after ingesting bacteria, and it takes only a few organisms to cause illness. A person is infectious from the time the diarrhea appears until the bacteria are no longer in the stool (about a month).

Food sources Milk and dairy products, poultry, mixed salads (tuna, potato, shrimp, macaroni, and chicken), and raw vegetables, mostly, but the bacteria can develop in any moist food that isn't thoroughly cooked. They multiply rapidly at room temperature.

Onset From eight hours to a week after consuming
   tainted food or beverages.
Symptoms Nausea and vomiting, diarrhea, stomach
   cramps, weakness, vision problems, headache, difficulty in swallowing. Children or those with weakened immune systems may have more serious diarrhea.
Diagnosis A culture of the stool will reveal the infection.
Treatment Most people recover on their own, but some
   may need fluids to offset dehydration. Antibiotics
   will help stop the diarrhea, although *Shigella* is becoming resistant to some drugs. Antidiarrhea medications should not be taken.
Prevention Confirmed cases must be reported to the
   local health department, which will begin an investi-
   gation and impose control measures in order to
   prevent large-scale outbreaks. Although several vac-
   cines have been tested, none has yet been licensed.
   The most important way to prevent the spread of this
   disease is to wash your hands carefully after using
   the toilet.

Staphylococcus Aureus

Staphylococcus aureus is one of the most common
sources of food poisoning in the United States, af-
fecting almost everyone at least once in his or her life.
This heat-resistant bacterium causes about 1.5 million
cases of food-borne illness in the United States each
year. Although the bacteria themselves are easily destroyed by high heat, they produce a toxin that is resistant to heat, refrigeration, and freezing and may be
found in a wide variety of foods. Poisoning with
this type of bacteria usually occurs after eating food

that has been kept warm for several hours before being served. Food may be contaminated by infected food handlers who touch their noses (where the germs are found) and then the food they prepare. This type of poisoning may be suspected when there has been only a brief interval between eating and the onset of symptoms.

Food sources Sandwiches, pastries, salty or cold meats, cheese, ice cream, cream-filled baked goods, dried beef, sausage, gravy, or raw milk.

Onset From one to six hours after eating contaminated food (the incubation period depends on the amount of food eaten and the susceptibility of the consumer).

Symptoms Salivation followed by nausea and vomiting, abdominal cramps, and diarrhea; in severe poisoning there is vomiting, diarrhea, and sometimes shock. Symptoms usually fade after five to six hours, although a few fatal cases have been reported.

Complications Complications and death are rare.

Treatment Because of significant loss of fluids after vomiting and diarrhea, the patient may require IV fluids.

Prevention Don't touch food during preparation, especially if you have a cold or any sort of skin lesion. Keep hot foods hot and cold foods cold. The best way to prevent this type of food poisoning is to refrigerate perishable foods adequately. While heat does destroy the bacteria, it does not destroy the heat-resistant toxin.

Streptococcus

These bacteria (Group A and Group D) may not commonly be thought of as a source of food-borne illness, but in fact they can contaminate a wide variety of foods left at room temperature. The bacteria get into the food most times because of poor hygiene, poor sanitary conditions, and ailing food handlers. Before the advent of milk pasteurization, Group A sore throats and scarlet fever were common (recently, salad bars have been implicated).

Food sources Group A strep: milk, ice cream, eggs, steamed lobster, ground ham, potato or egg salad, custard, rice pudding, shrimp salad.

Group D strep: sausage, evaporated milk, cheese, meat croquettes, meat pie, pudding, milk.

Onset Group A: onset within one to three days.

Group D: onset within two to thirty-six hours.

Symptoms Group A: septic sore throat, scarlet fever, blood poisoning.

Group D: diarrhea, cramps, nausea and vomiting, fever, chills, dizziness.

Diagnosis Group A: nasal and throat swabs.

Group D: stool and blood samples.

Treatment Antibiotics.

Complications Rare.

Vibrio Parahaemolyticus

Vibrio gastroenteritis is caused by eating fish or shellfish contaminated with *V. parahaemolyticus*. Sporadic outbreaks of this type of gastroenteritis have appeared in the United States, and the illness is very common in

Japan, where large outbreaks often occur. It appears when the bacteria attach themselves to a person's small intestine and secrete an as-yet-unidentified toxin.

Food sources Raw or improperly cooked contaminated fish and shellfish. Anyone who eats them is at risk, especially during the warmer months. Improper refrigeration of contaminated seafood allows the bacteria to grow, increasing the chance of infection.

Onset Between four and ninety-six hours after ingestion.

Symptoms Diarrhea, abdominal cramps, nausea and vomiting, headache, fever, and chills.

Diagnosis The organism can be cultured from a person's stool.

Treatment Drink plenty of fluids. In most cases, the infection will clear up by itself. Only a few cases require hospitalization and treatment with antibiotics.

Prognosis The illness is usually mild, although some people may need to be hospitalized.

Prevention Seafoods should be cooked at 160°F for at least 15 minutes, or until completely cooked.

Vibrio Vulnificus

This rare bacterium was first recognized as the cause of an unusually severe syndrome of food-borne illness called primary septicemia (blood poisoning) that can seriously affect people with an underlying disease. People at high risk for infection with serious consequences include those with liver disease, iron disorder (hemochromatosis), diabetes, cancer, HIV infection or AIDS, or long-term steroid use (such as chronic asthma patients). However, when ingested by healthy people, *V. vulnificus* causes only minor stomach discomfort.

While no major outbreaks have been reported, sporadic cases occur often. Florida reported thirty-eight cases of septicemia and seven cases of gastroenteritis from this bacterium between 1981 and 1987.

Food sources Raw or undercooked contaminated seafood such as oysters, clams, and crabs harvested in warm water, especially the Gulf of Mexico.

Onset Healthy patients become ill between twelve hours and a week after eating raw contaminated seafood.

Symptoms Gastrointestinal complaints.

Complications Blood clotting problems can occur.

Prognosis Among certain people—cancer patients, diabetics, the elderly, and those with weakened immune systems—the risk of serious illness rises sharply; their fatality rate is more than 50 percent.

Prevention People at high risk should avoid raw seafood.

Yersinia

The most recent *Yersinia* outbreak was in Georgia in 1988–89. Infection is often reported in young children. The CDC estimates individual *Yersinia* infections at about 17,000 cases a year.

Food sources Pork products, milk, oysters, fish, beef, lamb, and game.

Onset One to seven days.

Symptoms Acute diarrhea and fever, stomach pain that

may be mistaken for appendicitis, bloody diarrhea. Adults experience painful joints as well.

Treatment Antibiotics are effective and should be taken for up to seven days; serious illness may require hospitalization.

Complications Internal infection and arthritis.

Prognosis Mild to moderate infection that is usually self-limiting.

Prevention Don't consume raw pork or unpasteurized milk; maintain good kitchen-cleaning standards.

II. PARASITIC FOOD POISONING AND TOXIC SEAFOOD

A surprising number of parasites contaminate undercooked and raw fish and shellfish, and they can pose a health threat to anyone who eats them. The problem has intensified with the increasing popularity of sushi bars, raw bars, and international travel. Many infections are self-limiting, but some can be fatal if not treated. Parasitic infestations are especially a problem to anyone with a chronic underlying disease, such as AIDS.

The most common parasites that we can acquire from eating infected undercooked fish and shellfish are worms.

Toxins may also be produced as fish spoil (as in scombroid toxin) or as the by-products of toxic plankton (paralytic shellfish poisoning)—or they may be present naturally in the fish itself (tetrodotoxin).

Anisakis

The disorder anisakiasis is caused by a parasitic worm, *Anisakis simplex,* which infests small crustaceans eaten by many kinds of fish, dolphins, and whales. Fertilized eggs from the female parasite are eliminated by the host fish, and these develop into larvae that hatch in salt water.

Fewer than ten cases are diagnosed in the United States annually; however, experts suspect many cases go undiagnosed. Japan has the greatest number of cases because of the large amounts of raw fish eaten there. Anisakiasis is easily misdiagnosed as acute appendicitis, Crohn's disease, gastric ulcer, or gastrointestinal cancer.

Food sources Raw, undercooked, or insufficiently frozen fish and shellfish. Incidence is expected to increase with the increasing popularity of sushi and sashimi bars. The parasite can be found in raw herring as well as in sushi, sashimi, and seviche; host fish include cod, haddock, fluke, flounder, monkfish, and Pacific salmon.

Onset Symptoms may appear from one hour to two weeks after consuming raw or undercooked seafood.

Symptoms If the worm is not coughed up or passed into the bowels, it can penetrate the stomach and cause severe pain, nausea, and vomiting. In severe cases, the pain is akin to acute appendicitis, accompanied by nausea.

Diagnosis In North America, the infestation is usually diagnosed when the patient begins to feel a tingling or tickling sensation in the throat, and coughs up a worm. Otherwise, a physician may need to examine the inside of the person's stomach and the small intestine.

Treatment Surgically removing the worm(s) is the only known method of reducing the pain and eliminating the infestation.

Prevention You can kill the worms by cooking or freezing the fish. Marinating raw fish in lemon or vinegar doesn't kill all the harmful parasites (or bacteria) that the fish could contain. If you want to eat sushi, eat only at reputable restaurants and ask whether the fish was previously frozen (freezing reduces the risk of illness by killing larvae of parasites that might have been present in the raw fish).

Cryptosporidium

One of the more recently discovered types of food poisoning, cryptosporidiosis is a reportable disease caused by the protozoan *Cryptosporidium parvum*. This microbe infects cells lining the intestinal tract; it was not identified as a cause of human disease until 1976.

In 1993, a waterborne outbreak in Milwaukee sickened about 400,000 people, and the disease has been associated with diarrhea outbreaks in child care centers throughout the country. In 1994, 302 cases were reported to the New York State Department of Health.

Today it is a major threat to the U.S. water supply. Able to infect with as few as thirty oocysts, *Cryptosporidium* has been found in untreated surface water as well as in swimming pools, wading pools, hot tubs, ice cubes, fruits and vegetables, lakes, rivers, day care centers, and hospitals.

Experts estimate that 2 percent of the population in North America is infected, and that 80 percent of the population have had an infection in the past. In the United States, many outbreaks are never positively identified, and the number of cases that occur each year aren't well documented. Some immunity follows infection, but the degree to which immunity occurs is not clear.

This invisible parasite lives its entire life within the intestinal cells; it produces worms that are excreted in feces. The infectious worms can survive outside the human body for long periods of time, passing into food and drinking water, onto objects, and from hand to mouth.

Because cryptosporidiosis is transmitted by the fecal-oral route, the greatest risk comes from those infected people who have diarrhea, those with poor personal hygiene, and diapered children.

Food sources Contaminated water, vegetables fertilized with manure, unpasteurized milk, or any food touched by an infected person.

Onset One to twelve days after infection.

Symptoms Watery diarrhea together with stomach cramps, nausea and vomiting, fever, headache, and loss of appetite. Some people with the infection don't experience any symptoms at all. Healthy patients usually suffer with symptoms for only about two weeks.

Diagnosis The parasite may be detected during examination of the stool. If cryptosporidiosis is suspected, a specific lab test should be requested, since most labs don't yet routinely perform the necessary tests.

Treatment There is no standard treatment, but some patients may respond to some antibiotics. Intravenous fluids may be necessary, and antidiarrhea drugs may help.

Complications The person with an impaired immune system may have a severe and lasting illness; the resulting chronic diarrhea in this group can be fatal. Parasitic invasion of the lungs in these patients can also be fatal.

Prevention Unfortunately, chlorine does not kill the protozoan; drinking water must be filtered to eliminate it. Many municipal water systems do not have the resources to provide this type of filtration. To prevent further transmission, wash your hands often before and while you prepare food, especially if you change diapers or work around young children. Infected people should not prepare any food that will be eaten raw. Thoroughly wash fruits and vegetables before eating. Cattle are a source of infection, so don't drink unpasteurized milk or untreated, unfiltered water in other countries.

Cyclospora Cayetanensis

Another one-celled organism, called *Cyclospora cayetanensis*, causes symptoms similar to *Cryptosporidium* that were found in hundreds of residents of at least a dozen states in 1995. Like *Cryptosporidium*, *Cyclospora* pollutes water and taints food. The infection is spread by the fecal-oral route, both from person to person and via tainted water or food.

The United States is currently battling its fourth epidemic of *Cyclospora* infection, which began in the spring of 1996 and has included an outbreak in eleven states east of the Rocky Mountains in which a thousand people got sick from contaminated raspberries. Since the infection is fairly new, experts believe many cases are simply not diagnosed or reported. Your doctor must specifically request testing for *Cyclospora*; the lab test is not routine.

Food sources Some cases have been traced to contaminated strawberries, others to raspberries or mixed fruit. In other cases, experts can't find the original source of the infection.

Onset One to two weeks after infection.

Symptoms Diarrhea, nausea, and vomiting, with fever and stomach pain. Symptoms may be intermittent over the course of the disease, which can last for several weeks. While rarely fatal, untreated diarrhea can cause severe dehydration, which can be a serious health threat to very young children, very old people, and those with faulty immune systems. If not treated, symptoms may last for a few days to a month or more.

Diagnosis Special lab tests, which may require specimens over several days, can identify the parasite in stool.

Treatment A combination of two antibiotics can control the infection. Otherwise, rest and drink plenty of fluids.

Prevention Wash hands often, especially if you change diapers or work around young children. Thoroughly wash fruits and vegetables before eating. Infected people should not prepare food that is eaten raw. People in areas of high infection should boil water for one minute before using. The organism doesn't appear to be killed by iodine or chlorine, and can even elude filtration systems. The only thing that kills this parasite is boiling the water in which it lives.

Diphyllobothrium Latum

Diphyllobothriasis is caused by eating fish infested with a broad fish tapeworm *(Diphyllobothrium latum)*. Now uncommon in the United States, it was formerly often found in the Great Lakes area, where it was known as "Jewish disease" or "Scandinavian housewife's disease" because preparers of gefilte fish or fish balls tended to taste their food as they prepared it, before fish was fully cooked. The parasite is now supposedly absent from Great Lakes fish. Recently, however, cases have been reported on the West Coast.

Foods are not routinely analyzed for this parasite. In 1980 an outbreak involving four Los Angeles physicians occurred when the four ate sushi made of tuna, red snapper, and salmon. At the time of this outbreak, there was also a general increase in requests for niclosamide (the drug used to treat the infestation). Interviews of thirty-nine patients with similar symptoms at the time showed that thirty-two remembered eating salmon before becoming sick.

The disease is caused by parasitic flatworms and other members of this tapeworm family; the larva are often found in the viscera of freshwater and marine fish. After a person eats infected fish, an adult tapeworm between three and ten feet long grows in his or her small intestine; about a month later, the tapeworm begins to release more than a million eggs into the stool every day. Infection is usually limited to one worm.

Food sources Freshwater fish, or fish that migrate from salt water to fresh water for breeding, including pike, salmon, trout, whitefish, and turbot.

Onset About ten days after eating raw or undercooked fish.

Symptoms Many people don't have any symptoms, but others report a variety of minor complaints including distended abdomen, flatulence, nausea, headache, nervousness, weakness, cramping, and diarrhea. Some report a sensation that "something is moving inside." Those who are infected (usually people of Scandinavian heritage) may experience severe anemia caused by the tapeworm's absorption of vitamin B_{12}.

Diagnosis The disease is identified by finding eggs in the patient's feces.

Treatment Niclosamide or praziquantel will cure the infection.

Entamoeba Histolytica

Amoebic dysentery (amebiasis) is caused by the protozoan *Entamoeba histolytica* normally found in the human intestinal tract and feces. Anyone can get amebiasis, but it occurs most often among people who have just visited tropical or subtropical areas, and people in institutions.

The most dramatic outbreak in the United States was

during the Chicago World's Fair in 1933, when defective plumbing led to contaminated drinking water and one thousand cases (and fifty-eight deaths). More recently, outbreaks have been traced to food handlers, but there has been no single large outbreak.

Food sources The protozoa can be introduced to food and water through fecal contamination or when food handlers don't wash their hands.

Onset Within a few days to a few months after exposure (usually within two to four weeks).

Symptoms Symptoms include tenderness over the area of the colon or liver, loose morning stools, diarrhea, nervousness, weight loss, and fatigue.

Diagnosis Examination of stool under a microscope (several stool samples may be needed).

Treatment Specific antibiotics can treat amebiasis.

Complications The parasite can move on from the intestines and cause a more serious infection, such as a liver abscess, but death is rare.

Prevention Careful handwashing after using the rest room and proper disposal of sewage can prevent transmission of this parasite.

Giardia Lamblia

Giardia lamblia is a single-celled protozoan that is the most frequent cause of nonbacterial diarrhea in North America. You need to ingest only one cyst to become ill. The infestation is most often associated with contaminated water, often close to home. Recent outbreaks have been linked to public swimming pools;

while chlorine does kill the parasite, it takes about fifteen minutes. In that time, *Giardia* can enter the digestive tract of someone who swallows the contaminated pool water.

Giardiasis is most often transmitted from person to person by the fecal-oral route, transferring the parasites from hand to mouth. Five outbreaks have been traced to food contaminated by infected food handlers, and the disease is associated with poor hygiene and sanitation in day care centers. The organism flourishes in cool, moist conditions.

Giardiasis is more common in children than in adults, perhaps because many people seem to develop an immunity after one infection. *Giardia* is linked to 25 percent of cases of gastrointestinal disease; about 2 percent of the population is believed to be infected at any one time. The disease is common in day care centers. Major outbreaks are associated with contaminated water systems that don't use sand filtration, or that have a defective filtration system.

Food sources Contaminated water, contaminated raw vegetables, food handled by infected workers.

Onset About a week after ingesting the parasite.

Symptoms Greasy diarrhea, gas, stomach cramps, fatigue, and weight loss. Some people may not have any symptoms at all. The infection usually passes in a week or two, although some people suffer for months.

Treatment Flagyl is effective in treating the infection.

Complications Severe infection may damage parts of the digestive tract.

Prevention Wash hands after using the toilet, changing diapers, and so on. Chlorinated water may not kill the *Giardia* cysts. Purify untreated water while camping by boiling for one full minute. If you suspect foreign water is tainted, stick to beverages made with boiled water (coffee or tea), or drink bottled beverages without ice. Avoid raw produce that can't be peeled.

Nanophyetus

Nanophyetiasis is caused by eating seafood tainted with worms (*Nanophyetus salmincola* or *N. schikhobalowi*), which are transmitted as larvae that embed themselves in the flesh of freshwater fish. There have been no reports of massive outbreaks; the only scientific report has been twenty people in Oregon who came down with the disease. However, the condition is endemic in Russia, where the infection rate is reported to be more than 90 percent and growing.

Food sources North American cases were all associated with raw, smoked, and underprocessed salmon and steelhead.

Symptoms Diarrhea, usually accompanied by stomach discomfort and nausea; a few people reported weight loss and fatigue.

Diagnosis The disease is diagnosed by finding the eggs in feces. However, it's hard to tell the difference between these eggs and those of another parasite *(Diphyllobothrium latum)*.

Treatment Treatment with niclosamide or bithionol appears to cure the infection.

Prevention Be cautious about eating salmon from areas
of high infestation.

Toxoplasma Gondii

Toxoplasmosis is caused by the parasite *Toxoplasma
gondii*, which is transmitted to humans via undercooked meat (among other ways). It's most serious in
pregnant women: 7 percent of the fetuses have minor
abnormalities, 3 percent have severe damage. Highest
risk occurs if the mother has been infected during the
first six months of pregnancy.

Food sources Undercooked beef, mutton, or lamb from
an infected animal, or unpasteurized milk from an infected goat; water contaminated with cat feces. Humans aren't infectious to each other.
Onset Between five and twenty days after exposure.
Symptoms Clinical signs are usually mild, with a slight
swelling of lymph nodes along with a low-grade
fever, fatigue, sore throat, or slight body rash. High-
risk individuals may experience severe symptoms
involving multiple organs.
Diagnosis Blood tests reveal the parasite.
Treatment Severe cases are treated with sulfonamides
and pyrimethamine; healthy nonpregnant young adults
don't need to be treated.
Complications In infants born to infected mothers,
complications include eye problems, water on the
brain, jaundice, vomiting, fever, convulsions, or mental retardation. High-risk individuals may have pneu-
monia or heart infection, and may die.

Prevention High-risk people should avoid eating raw or undercooked meat.

Trichinella Spiralis

Trichinosis is a type of potentially fatal food poisoning caused by the larvae of a parasitic worm; once ingested, the larvae develop in the intestinal wall, migrate through the body, and penetrate the muscles. Most recently, *Trichinella spiralis* been found in undercooked pork in Iowa in 1990. Partial immunity may follow an infection.

Routine inspection of carcasses for *Trichinella* organisms is not performed in the United States because the disease is on the decline; also, irradiation of pork carcasses can eradicate the larvae.

Food sources Undercooked pork, the meat of wild animals and marine mammals, and horsemeat.

Onset Between one and seven weeks after eating contaminated food.

Symptoms Diarrhea, fever, sore muscles, and swollen eyelids. These symptoms are followed by pain and bleeding in the eyes, thirst, chills, sweating, and weakness. Symptoms may last for months.

Diagnosis Blood tests can confirm the infection by detecting antibodies to the larvae, or a muscle biopsy can reveal the larvae themselves.

Treatment Mebendazole is an effective treatment; failure to treat the infection could be fatal. Bed rest is recommended to prevent relapse.

Complications In severe cases, there may be heart and neurological problems that can progress to fatal heart failure, either in the first two weeks after infection, or between the fourth and eighth week.

Prevention Cook all pork products and wild game completely (to an internal temperature of at least 160°F) at 350°F for 35 minutes per pound. Pork should be a gray color on the inside, with no visible pink. Storing infected meat in a freezer with a temperature no higher than −13°F for ten days will also kill the parasite. Pork or pork products should never be eaten raw, and even smoked or salted meat may still have organisms. Pork should not be ground in the same grinder as other meats, and the grinder used should be well cleaned afterward.

Toxic Shellfish

Seafood contaminated with toxins may look and taste normal, but normal cooking methods don't affect the toxins. State shellfish screening programs test shellfish for the presence of these toxins, and monitor the safety of shellfish harvest beds. However, people who catch their own shellfish from unapproved beds are at risk for a variety of toxic infections.

Some types of plankton eaten by shellfish along the North American coasts produce a toxin known as saxitoxin. These plankton multiply rapidly during the warm summer months; because their color is pink or red, the phenomenon has come to be called red tide. When people eat shellfish contaminated with the toxin, they can become very sick or die. It's not possible to build up immunity by becoming exposed to sublethal doses; in fact, in some cases the substance is so toxic that even one contaminated shellfish can be fatal if eaten. Remember: this is why clams, oysters, and mussels are not sold during months without an "R" (the summer months).

Shellfish poisoning caused by these toxic plankton comes in four forms: paralytic shellfish poisoning (PSP), neurotoxic shellfish poisoning (NSP), amnesic shellfish poisoning (ASP), and diarrheic shellfish poisoning (DSP). Each has quite different etiology, symptoms, and prognosis for recovery, but of the four, PSP is by far the most serious. The other three types of toxic shellfish poisoning are caused by twenty different toxins related to saxitoxin. The true incidence of these shellfish poisonings is not known; it is believed that many cases aren't reported.

Paralytic Shellfish Poisoning (PSP)

While shellfish by themselves are not poisonous, they can become contaminated by bacteria from their environment, and pass it on to humans when the shellfish are eaten. Most cases of PSP, the most serious form of shellfish poisoning caused by toxic plankton, have occurred when people ate raw shellfish. Even so, cooking will not destroy the toxin.

Paralytic shellfish poisoning was recorded as early as 1689, and outbreaks have been recorded many times since then. One of the highest concentrations of PSP in the world is reported to be in shellfish in southeast Alaska. Most victims of PSP are people who have gathered shellfish for their own consumption. Traditionally, it has been considered a danger associated only with shellfish harvested in cold water, but the incidence in tropical areas has been increasing.

Food sources Oysters, clams, cockles, and mussels are particularly prone to contamination because of their respiratory systems, which pump water across the gills to isolate plankton for their food. Crustacean shellfish (such as lobsters) only very rarely transmit PSP. In mussels, toxins are concentrated in the digestive glands and toxicity is usually lost within weeks, but the Alaskan butter clam can remain toxic for up to two years. However, the part of the mollusk that humans generally eat—the white meat, without the digestive glands—stores fairly small amounts of toxin.

Onset Signs of poisoning develop within five to thirty minutes after eating contaminated crabs, clams, or mussels.

Symptoms Gradual paralysis and trembling, with nausea, vomiting, and diarrhea. Later on, there may be shortness of breath, dry mouth, a choking feeling, confused or slurred speech, and lack of coordination. Eating even a tiny amount of contaminated shellfish can be fatal, and survival usually depends on how much has been consumed.

Treatment There is no known antidote for shellfish poisoning caused by saxitoxin and no drug has proven effective, so treatment is only supportive. CPR may be needed as first aid.

Prognosis If the victim survives the first twelve hours, prognosis for complete recovery (within a few days to two weeks) is good. However, between 8.5 and 23.2 percent of PSP poisonings are fatal.

Prevention You can't tell just by looking at the water whether toxic plankton are present. If you're not sure if the seafood you're eating is toxin-free, avoid eating it if it's been harvested from an area with a high incidence of the poison. To prevent outbreaks, state health departments test samples of susceptible shellfish for toxin during certain times of the year. Affected growing areas are quarantined, and sale of shellfish is prohibited. Warnings are posted in shellfish growing areas, on beaches, and in the news. You can't eliminate PSP from shellfish by cooking or freezing; even when pressure-cooked at 250°F for fifteen minutes, the shellfish remain toxic.

Neurotoxic Shellfish Poisoning (NSP)

Neurotoxic shellfish poisoning attacks the nervous system and includes both stomach and neurological problems.

Food source NSP is associated with shellfish harvested along the coasts of Florida, North Carolina, and the Gulf of Mexico.

Onset Symptoms occur within a few minutes to a few hours after eating contaminated shellfish.

Symptoms Tingling and numb lips, tongue, and throat; muscular aches; dizziness; reversal of sensations; diarrhea; and vomiting. Symptoms last between a few hours and a few days. Recovery is complete with very few aftereffects; no fatalities have been reported.

Prevention Monitoring programs can prevent human infection. Eat only shellfish from reportable sources and approved beds.

Amnesic Shellfish Poisoning (ASP)

Amnesic shellfish poisoning was first identified in 1987 in an outbreak that killed three and sickened more than a hundred in Canada.

Food source ASP is associated primarily with mussels.

Onset Symptoms appear within twenty-four hours and neurological symptoms follow within forty-eight hours.

Symptoms ASP can be life-threatening, causing stomach problems (vomiting, diarrhea, and abdominal pain). In severe cases, neurological problems (confusion, memory loss, disorientation, seizure, and coma) also appear. The poisoning is especially serious for older patients and may appear to resemble Alzheimer's disease. All known fatalities have occurred in elderly patients.

Prevention Eat only shellfish from reportable sources and approved beds.

Diarrheic Shellfish Poisoning (DSP)

While diarrheic shellfish poisoning has not been confirmed in the United States, the organisms that produce the poison are found in U.S. waters and an outbreak has been confirmed in eastern Canada.

Food sources DSP is associated primarily with mussels, oysters, and scallops.

Onset This diarrhea-causing shellfish poisoning begins as early as within thirty minutes to two or three hours, depending on the amount of tainted shellfish eaten.

Symptoms Diarrhea may last as long as two or three days, but recovery is complete with no aftereffects and the disease is not usually life-threatening.

Cigua Toxin

Ciguatera poisoning occurs after eating any of more than three hundred species of fish that may contain cigua toxin; the toxin is found in greatest concentration in internal organs, but it can't be detected by inspection, taste, or smell. The fish are toxic at those times of the year when they ingest a certain type of plankton, which produce the cigua toxin—an odorless, tasteless poison that can't be destroyed by either heating or freezing.

Ciguatera poisoning occurs most often in the Caribbean islands, Florida, Hawaii, and the Pacific Islands. Recently, 129 cases were reported over a two-year period in Dade County, Florida, alone. It appears to be occurring more often, probably because of the increased demand for seafood around the world and the resurgence of the toxin in edible fish. Experts believe this type of poisoning is underreported because it is usually not fatal and symptoms don't last long.

Isolated instances of ciguatera poisoning have occurred along the eastern United States coast, from South Florida to Vermont. Hawaii, the U.S. Virgin Islands, and Puerto Rico also report sporadic cases.

Food sources Cigua toxin is usually found in larger coral reef fish, including barracuda, snapper, amberjack, surgeonfish, sea bass, and grouper. Other species of warm-water fish, such as mackerel or triggerfish, may be contaminated. Not all fish of a given species or from a given locality will be toxic at the same time.

Symptoms Both stomach and neurologic symptoms, with a curious type of sensory reversal, so that picking up a cold glass would cause a burning-hot sensation. Other symptoms include a tingling sensation in the lips and mouth, followed by numbness, nausea, vomiting, abdominal cramps, weakness, headache, vertigo, paralysis, convulsions, and skin rash; coma and death from respiratory paralysis occur in about 12 percent of cases. Subsequent episodes of ciguatera poisoning may be more severe. Ciguatera poisoning is usually self-limiting, and subsides within several days.

Complications Sometimes the neurological symptoms may persist for weeks or months. Occasionally symptoms have lasted for several years, or patients have relapsed. These relapses may be associated with alcohol consumption or dietary changes. Rarely, death occurs from respiratory or heart failure.

Treatment Effective antidotes are available.

Prevention The only way to prevent this infection is to avoid tropical reef fish, since there is no easy way to routinely measure the toxin in any seafood product before eating.

Scombroid Toxin

Scombroid poisoning is caused by eating spoiled fish (especially tuna or mahimahi). However, eating any food that contains the right amount of amino acids and bacteria may lead to scombroid poisoning. Even though this is one of the most common types of fish poisoning in the United States, many cases aren't reported. While anyone can contract scombroid poisoning, symptoms are especially serious in older people and those taking certain medications (such as isoniazid).

Food sources Fish implicated in scombroid poisoning include bluefish, sardines, mackerel, amberjack, and abalone, but many other products can also cause these toxic effects, including Swiss cheese.

Onset Symptoms may appear immediately after eating the tainted food or up to thirty minutes after.

Symptoms First comes a tingling or burning sensation in the mouth, a rash on the upper body, and dropping blood pressure, with headaches and itchy skin. These may be followed by nausea and vomiting, with diarrhea. Older or chronically ill people may need to be hospitalized. The duration of the illness is usually about three hours, although it may last for several days.

Prevention Neither cooking, canning, nor freezing can reduce the toxic effect, and you can't smell or taste a problem. Chemical testing is the only reliable way to evaluate the product.

Tetrodotoxin

The puffer fish *(Arothron meleagris)* is an exotic food fish considered a delicacy in Japan, where it is known as *fugu*. However, this fish can cause poisoning if improperly prepared and cooked, and is considered to be one of the most poisonous fish in the world, with a 60 percent fatality rate even with treatment. There have been hundreds of deaths in Japan; at least three have been reported in Florida. Puffer fish are most toxic just before and during their reproductive season, because of the interaction between gonad activity and toxicity, although individual fish of the same species found in different locations at the same time could vary widely in their toxicity.

In Japan, cooks and restaurants that serve puffer fish must have a special license to prepare this often-deadly dish. Usually eaten only during the winter months (not its reproductive season), puffer fish is still the primary cause of death from food poisoning in Japan.

The poison in the puffer fish is tetrodotoxin, a basic compound that does not deactivate when heated and that carries a high fatality rate when eaten.

Onset Symptoms begin within minutes to hours after eating improperly prepared fish.

Symptoms Numbness and tingling beginning in the extremities and spreading over the body, together with a feeling of floating. This is followed by nausea and vomiting, and other gastrointestinal symptoms. Paralysis follows in an ascending pattern, which begins as the victim finds it difficult to breathe, then progresses to coma, convulsions, respiratory arrest, and death. The first twenty-four hours after ingestion are critical.

Treatment There is no antidote to tetrodotoxin and there is great controversy over the relative benefits of the administration of atropine, edrophonium, or pyridostigmine. Otherwise, treatment is supportive.

III. VIRAL FOOD POISONING

Hepatitis A

"Hepatitis" is simply a term that refers to any inflammation of the liver; the inflammation is generally caused by a virus. The hardy hepatitis A virus is the most common type of all the alphabet hepatitis viruses, and is transmitted via contaminated food and water. Unlike many other viruses, it can live for more than a month at room temperature on kitchen countertops, children's toys, and other surfaces, and it can be maintained indefinitely in frozen foods and ice.

In 1994, 22,000 Americans were reported to have hepatitis A, but thousands of cases go unreported. While there is not a typical "season" for hepatitis A, it tends to occur in cycles. Mass food-borne contaminations have included frozen strawberries in Michigan, imported lettuce in Louisville, slushy beverages in Alaska, restaurant iced tea in North Carolina, raw oysters in Florida, unidentified food in a Washington restaurant chain, north Georgia frozen strawberries, Montana frozen strawberries, and Baltimore shellfish.

The virus causes an estimated 130,000 infections and 100 deaths each year. More than 40 percent of healthy adults in the United States are immune to hepatitis A as a result of previous infection. The disease occurs most often among school-age children and young adults. It is spread when people eat food or drink water contaminated with the hepatitis A virus, and then the virus multiplies in the body, is passed in the feces, and finally is carried on the infected person's hands and spread by direct contact, or by others' eating food or drink handled by that person.

Food sources Shellfish (especially oysters), other raw or undercooked food, well water contaminated by improperly treated sewage.

Onset Incubation period ranges from fifteen to fifty days.

Symptoms One-quarter of all people with hepatitis A won't have any symptoms; a few young children may have a low fever and achiness, but rarely jaundice. Children over age twelve may get much sicker, with fever (100°F to 104°F), extreme tiredness, weakness, nausea, stomach upset, pain in the upper right side of the abdomen, and appetite loss. Within a few days, a yellowish tinge appears in the skin and whites of the eyes. Urine will be darker than usual and the stool light-colored. Once the jaundice appears, patients begin to feel better.

Diagnosis Blood tests showing antibodies to hepatitis A are the best diagnosis. Symptoms of hepatitis A are so similar to those of other diseases that a doctor needs a test to make the correct diagnosis.

Treatment There is no drug treatment for hepatitis A. While symptoms appear, patients should rest and eat well: a low-fat, high-carbohydrate diet of easily digested foods in small amounts (good choices are crackers, noodles, rice, and soup). Antinausea medicine and acetaminophen may be prescribed.

Complications Rarely, hepatitis A develops into fulminant hepatitis, in which the liver cells are completely destroyed. As the liver function stops, toxic substances build up and affect the brain, causing lethargy, confusion, combativeness, stupor, and coma. This can often lead to death, although with aggressive treatment the patient may live. If the victim does not die, the liver is able to regenerate and resume function and the brain recovers.

Prognosis Hepatitis A is less serious than other types of hepatitis, and causes only temporary liver damage, which is reversed as the body produces antibodies. Most people recover in a few weeks without any complications. However, it can occasionally be fatal; about one hundred people die each year.

Prevention To inactivate the virus, food must be heated at 185°F for 1 minute. It is difficult to test water for hepatitis A, but treated municipal or county water supplies are safe. Patients are most infectious in the two weeks before symptoms develop. Food handlers who know they are infected should not work until they are past the infectious stage, which ends one week after one first becomes jaundiced. Even though federal regulations and postings of contaminated water offer some protection, there is still a risk of contracting hepatitis A when eating raw shellfish.

Norwalk Virus

The most common source of viral contamination in shellfish is the Norwalk virus, which can taint raw or improperly cooked food that has been in contact with water contaminated by human excrement. The disease is mild and self-limiting.

Among recent outbreaks have been an incident with Gulf Coast oysters in Louisiana in 1994, and a multistate outbreak associated with oysters in Florida.

Food sources Shellfish and salad ingredients are most often implicated in outbreaks; eating raw or poorly steamed clams and oysters poses a high risk of infection. Foods other than shellfish can be contaminated by ailing food handlers.

Onset Symptoms begin one or two days after eating.

Symptoms Fever, weakness, appetite loss, headache, diarrhea, nausea, vomiting, and stomach pain. Severe illness is very rare.

Complications None.

Prognosis Norwalk virus infection is usually a mild, self-limiting condition that lasts for only one or two days.

Prevention Cook shellfish for at least 4 minutes at 194°F. Patients with diarrhea or vomiting should not prepare food.

IV. FUNGI

Aflatoxins

Mycotoxicosis is a type of poisoning caused by fungus-derived metabolites found on certain kinds of food. Ever since the Middle Ages, thousands of people have died from various types of mycotoxins, but it was a 1960 epidemic among turkeys in England that spurred a worldwide research effort to track down the vast number of toxic compounds derived from fungi. Among the most widespread of these fungal contaminations are the aflatoxins. Aflatoxin is a cancer-causing by-product of the *Aspergillus flavus* mold; the mold grows in the warm, humid climate of the southeastern United States, but it can also appear elsewhere when rain falls on corn and wheat left in the field to dry. Aflatoxin-producing mold can even grow on plants damaged by insects or drought, poor nutrition, or unseasonable temperatures. Aflatoxins are more common in poor-quality cereals and nuts; while most of these low-grade products don't enter the human food market, they are sold as animal feed, which can go on to contaminate animal products (such as meat and milk). For this reason, cottonseed meal (a product often contaminated with high levels of aflatoxin) is banned for use as an animal feed. Cottonseed oil, however, rarely contains aflatoxin, since the toxin sticks to the hulls of the seeds.

Aflatoxin has been called the most potent natural carcinogen known to humans. Still, scientists know very little about why or how the aflatoxins are produced by the mold.

While the way agricultural products are stored can affect the mold's growth, the length of time of such storage is also important; the longer agricultural products are stored in bins, the greater the chance that environmental conditions favorable to aflatoxin production will be created. Stored nuts or seeds might accidentally get wet or the storage bin might not facilitate drying quickly enough to stop the mold from growing.

Food sources Peanuts, corn, wheat, rice, cottonseed, barley, soybeans, Brazil nuts, pistachios, grains, tree nuts, cottonseed meal, meat, eggs, milk, powdered dry milk, baby food, chicken.

Symptoms Aflatoxin can cause acute poisoning; severe liver disease has been detected in those who ingest highly contaminated food; and children exhibit symptoms similar to Reye's syndrome (fever, vomiting, coma, and convulsions) after exposure.

Complication Aflatoxin is believed to cause liver cancer.

Prevention Consumers should never eat a moldy or shriveled food (especially grains or peanuts) and should be cautious about eating unroasted peanuts sold in bulk. Pasteurization, sterilization, and spray-dry processing techniques can substantially reduce aflatoxin contamination of dried milk. Because the mold is sometimes difficult to see, all susceptible crops are subject to routine testing in the United States, but it isn't possible to detect aflatoxin with 100 percent accuracy.

V. CONTAMINANTS

Chlorinated Compounds and Mercury

As discussed in Chapter 6, "Safe Seafood," fatty fish like salmon, bluefish, and herring are vulnerable to chlorinated compounds such as PCBs (polychlorinated biphenyls) and the insecticide DDT, which linger in the body for years. Very minute quantities of these substances in the water will produce very high concentrations in fish.

Mercury poisoning occurs through the contamination of fish in lakes and streams throughout the United States as a result of extensive agricultural fungicide and pesticide use, and the industrial by-products of chlorine production. Current estimates suggest up to 10,000 tons of mercury infiltrate the sea each year;

once in the water, it enters the food chain, where it is converted into organic methyl mercury, one of the most toxic substances known to man.

The presence of sewage in the water facilitates this deadly conversion. Contaminated bacteria living in mud is eaten by plankton, which are in turn eaten by fish. Methyl mercury seems to affect women more than men, and children and infants most of all.

The first cases of poisoning by contaminated fish occurred in Japan in 1953 and 1970, when more than 121 cases—and 46 deaths—were reported. At that time, methyl mercury chloride flowed directly into the bay and nearby river from a manufacturing plant. Nearly all fish contain trace amounts of methyl mercury. In areas of the United States where there is industrial mercury pollution, fish may have very high levels of contamination. However, the top ten seafood species (including shrimp, clams, crab, and canned tuna) are not subject to a risk of serious contamination.

Food sources Pike, pickerel, perch, walleye, muskie, white bass, swordfish, tuna, and shark.

Symptoms Mercury does not readily break down in the body, and can take months to be excreted. In addition, it can pass easily through the blood-brain barrier, irreversibly damaging brain cells; it also crosses the placenta and builds up in the fetal brain and blood. After weeks, months, or years of eating contaminated fish, methyl mercury poisoning affects the central nervous system, causing numbness or tingling of mouth, lips, tongue, and extremities;

visual disturbances; hearing problems; speech disorders; difficulty swallowing; weakness; fatigue; concentration problems; emotional changes and instability; inability to write, read, or remember simple things; and stumbling gait. In severe cases, it can lead to coma and death.

Diagnosis Methyl mercury can be detected in blood and hair samples.

Treatment Cheating agents, such as dimercaprol, are used to treat mercury poisoning and its symptoms.

Prognosis All forms of mercury are toxic to humans, but methyl mercury is especially of concern because our bodies have a less-well-developed defense mechanism against this toxin. In milder cases of mercury poisoning, impaired motor skills and dulled senses of touch, taste, and sight are reversible if exposure is stopped. However, extremely severe cases of poisoning can be fatal.

Prevention You can prevent mercury poisoning by eating a variety of fish, not just one kind, and by eating high-risk fish (such as swordfish) no more than once a week. Pregnant women should avoid eating swordfish more than once a month. Consumption advice is unnecessary for the top ten seafood species (canned tuna, shrimp, pollock, salmon, cod, catfish, clams, flatfish, crabs, and scallops), which make up about 80 percent of the seafood market.

If you suspect food poisoning of any kind, call your doctor immediately!

Glossary

Aluminum foil: Mostly aluminum wrap that works well in the refrigerator or freezer; one side is shiny, the other dull. It doesn't matter which side touches the food.

Antibacterial cleaner: A cleanser designed to clean surfaces and kill bacteria at the same time.

Antiseptic: A germicide intended for use on human skin or tissue (not objects). Antiseptics include alcohol, iodine, povidone-iodine (Betadine), hydrogen peroxide, chlorhexidine, and hexachlorophene (pHisoHex).

Bacteria: Single-celled microbes that multiply by dividing in two, and can be carried by water, wind, insects, plants, animals, and people. Among other things, bacteria survive in room-temperature foods.

Boil-in bag: A sealed container made of heat-resistant material designed to hold a food product and permit the consumer to bring bag and product to boiling.

Cross-contamination: The transfer of harmful substances or disease-causing organisms to food by hands, contaminated surfaces, sponges, dish towels, or utensils that touch raw food. Cross-contamination can also occur when raw food touches or drips onto cooked food.

Dehydration: Loss of water from body tissues, often as the result of severe vomiting or diarrhea.

Detergent: A preparation containing phosphates or other agents that are good for general cleaning. Household detergents or cleansers are not disinfectants and do not kill germs.

Disinfectant: A chemical germicide used to disinfect surfaces. Most disinfectants must not be used on human skin. Low-level disinfectants include alcohol, ammonium (used in many household disinfectants), chlorine, or hydrogen peroxide.

Disinfection: The elimination of most germs on surfaces.

Food-borne illness: An infection (also known as food poisoning) that is carried or transmitted by contaminated food.

Food irradiation: The treatment of food by ionizing radiation to slow down ripening or spoiling; it won't increase radioactivity level in food.

Freezer paper: White paper coated on one side with plastic to help keep air out of frozen food, protecting against freezer burn and loss of moisture.

Fungi: A group of organisms that include molds and yeasts.

Gastroenteritis: Inflammation of the stomach and intestines, usually due to infection by viruses or bacteria or food-poisoning toxins.

Germ: Any disease-causing microorganism, including bacteria, viruses, and fungi.

Mycotoxins: Toxins produced by fungi.

Oven cooking bags: Bags (and ties) made from heat-resistant nylon; they can be used in a microwave oven or conventional oven (at no higher than 400° F).

Parasite: Any organism that lives in or on another living organism.

Pasteurization: The process of applying heat (usually to milk or cheese) for a certain amount of time to kill bacteria.

Plankton: Tiny free-floating plants eaten by larger shellfish. Toxic forms of plankton (dinoflagellates) can be a source of shellfish poisoning.

Produce bags (in store): Usually made from polyethylene or other plastic film used for consumer in-store packaging of fruits and vegetables. They are not used in cooking, since the thin plastic could melt or burn.

Protozoa: A group of microscopic single-celled animals, some of which can cause disease.

Spore: Small reproductive body produced by plants and microorganisms.

Sterilization: A means of rendering objects free of microorganisms that would otherwise cause disease.

Toxic: Poisonous.

Toxins: Poisons that are products of living organisms; they may be produced by microorganisms, carried by fish, or released by plants. They include the toxin produced by *Clostridium botulinum*, which causes botulism, and the scombroid toxin found in some fish, such as tuna or mackerel, when they are poorly refrigerated.

Virus: The smallest, simplest life form known.

Waxed paper: A triple-waxed tissue paper made with food-safe paraffin wax that is forced into the pores of the paper and spread over the outside as a coating.

Appendix A

Hotlines

Most major food companies list 800 numbers on their labels, in case you have any question about an item.

HEPATITIS

Hepatitis C Helpline
415-834-4100

MEATS AND POULTRY

Armour-Swift-Eckrich
3131 Woodcreek Drive
Downers Grove, IL 60515
800-325-7424

Consumer-relations staffers answer questions on storage of products; weekdays, 8:30 A.M. to 4:30 P.M. CT.

Butterball Turkey Talk Line
Downers Grove, IL
800-323-4848

The staff can talk you through the preparation of a complete turkey dinner with all the trimmings. Open from November through Christmas, weekdays, 8 A.M. through 8 P.M. CT; open 6 A.M. through 6 P.M. Thanksgiving Day.

CDC Foodborne Disease Hotline
404-332-4597

Recorded messages in English and Spanish twenty-four hours a day.

Empire Kosher
River Road
Mifflintown, PA 17059
800-367-4734

Consumer-relations staffers answer questions about kosher processing, poultry handling, and preparation; they can also provide cooking directions.

Hormel Foods
2 Hormel Place
Austin, MN 55912
800-523-4635

Consumer-affairs staff provides recipes for and nutrient composition of Hormel products and handle complaints; weekdays, 8 A.M. to 4 P.M. CT.

Nutrition Hotline
American Dietetic Association
Chicago, IL
800-366-1655

Registered dieticians answer food- and nutrition-
related questions; taped nutrition messages available
twenty-four hours a day.

Tyson–Holly Farms and Weaver
Springdale, AK
800-233-6332

Staffers handle questions on safe handling and preparation of poultry products.

USDA Meat and Poultry Hotline
800-535-4555

Answers to questions about meat and poultry contamination, grading, and proper storage procedures; weekdays, 10 A.M. to 4 P.M. ET.

SEAFOOD

Seafood Safety Hotline
800-FDA-4010

Recorded messages on seafood purchasing, storage,
handling, labeling, and nutrition, and economic fraud;
twenty-four hours a day. To speak to an operator, call
weekdays between noon and 4 P.M. ET.

WATER

International Bottled Water Association
800-WATER-11

EPA Safe Drinking Water Hotline
800-426-4791
http://www.epa.gov/opptintr/lead/index.html

To speak to an operator, call weekdays, between 9:00 A.M. and 5:30 P.M. ET.

National Lead Information Center
800-424-LEAD
http://www.epa.gov/lead/nlic.htm

APPENDIX B

For More Information . . .

DETOXIFICATION INFORMATION AND SUPPLEMENTS

For a complete array of pesticide and industrial chemical analyses for blood, urine, and body tissues:

AccuChem Laboratories
990 North Bowser Road, Suite 800
Richardson, TX 75081
800-451-0116
972-234-5412

Pacific Toxicology
1545 Pontious Avenue
Los Angeles, CA 90025
310-479-4911

For information on a structured clinical detox program, contact:

HealthMed
5501 Power Inn Road, Suite 140
Sacramento, CA 95820
916-924-8060

E. COLI

The Brianne Kiner Foundation
P.O. Box 1053
Edmonds, WA 98020

FOOD ADDITIVES

Food Additives: A Shopper's Guide to What's Safe and What's Not

Pocket-sized book listing 600 common food additives classified according to safety and allergic reactions; send $4.95 to:
  Dr. Christine Hoza Farlow
  365 West Second Avenue, Suite 102
  Escondido, CA 92025

FOOD POISONING

"Who, Why, When, and Where of Food Poisons"
U.S. Food and Drug Administration
HFE-88
5600 Fishers Lane
Rockville, MD 20857

Chart identifying the more common sources of food poisoning and outlining how to prevent food contamination. Free in single quantities.

FOOD SAFETY

American Public Health Association
1015 Fifteenth Street NW
Washington, DC 20005
202-789-5600

Food Marketing Institute
800 Connecticut Avenue NW, Suite 500
Washington, DC 20006
202-452-8444

Microban Products Company
11515 Vanstory Drive, Suite 10
Huntersville, NC 28078
704-875-0806

Public Voice for Food and Health Policy
1101 Fourteenth Street NW, Suite 710
Washington, DC 20005
202-347-6200
http://www.publicvoice.org/pvoice.html

Public Voice for Food and Health Policy is a national, nonprofit research and analysis organization that looks at food and agriculture issues from a consumer perspective. It promotes a safer, healthier, and more affordable food supply for all Americans.

GOVERNMENT REGULATION

Centers for Disease Control and Prevention (CDC)
1600 Clifton Road NE
Atlanta, GA 30333
888-232-6789

Food Safety and Inspection Service (FSIS)
Room 1175, South Building
1400 Independence Avenue SW
Washington, DC 20250
202-720-7943

The public health agency in the USDA responsible for ensuring that meat, poultry, and egg products are safe and accurately labeled.

National Institute of Allergy and Infectious Diseases
National Institutes of Health
9000 Rockville Pike
Building 31, Room 7A32
Bethesda, MD 20892
301-496-4000

U.S. Food and Drug Administration
HFE-88
5600 Fishers Lane
Rockville, MD 20857
301-443-3380

The FDA is the primary consumer health protection agency of the federal government responsible for ensuring that food is safe. Its toxicology research is designed to provide data to strengthen the scientific base for assessing risk or safety.

HELICOBACTER PYLORI

The Helicobacter Foundation
P.O. Box 7965
Charlottesville, VA 22906
http://www.helico.com/

HEPATITIS

American Liver Foundation
1425 Pompton Avenue
Cedar Grove, NJ 07009
973-256-2550

INTERNATIONAL

World Health Organization
Avenue Appia
CH 1211 Geneva 27
Switzerland

MEAT

American Meat Institute
1700 North Moore Street, Suite 1600
Arlington, VA 22209
703-841-2400

National Livestock and Meat Board
44 North Michigan Avenue
Chicago, IL 60611

PESTICIDE REFORM

Mothers and Others for Pesticide Limits
P.O. Box 96641
Washington, DC 20090

National Coalition Against Misuse of Pesticides
701 East Street SE, Suite 200
Washington, DC 20003
202-543-5450

Disseminates information, helps grassroots groups
working to change pesticide laws; publishes newsletter.

Natural Resources Defense Council
71 Stevenson Street, Suite 1825
San Francisco, CA 94105
415-777-0220

Produces reports on pesticides.

Northwest Coalition for Alternatives to Pesticides
P.O. Box 1393
Eugene, OR 97440
541-344-5044

Five-state coalition fighting the U.S. Forest Service on
herbicide spraying; publishes the *Journal of Pesticide
Reform*.

Pesticide Action Network
North America Regional Center
49 Paul Street, Suite 500
San Francisco, CA 94102
415-981-1771

Worldwide organization of people and groups opposed
to the proliferation of pesticides.

SEAFOOD

Cigua-Check Kit
Oceanit Test Systems, Inc.
1100 Alakea Street, 31st Floor
Honolulu, HI 96813
808-539-2345
http://www.cigua.com

The only kit commercially available that detects cigua
toxin in fish.

"Get Hooked on Seafood Safety"
Consumer Information Center
Department 526Z
Pueblo, CO 81009

Write for this free brochure.

TRAVEL

Centers for Disease Control and Prevention
Health Information for International Travel

The "Yellow Book" is being revised; the new 1999 version will soon be available. The book can be downloaded or ordered for $20.00 by calling 202-512-1800 and requesting stock #017-023-00197-3.

Traveling Healthy
108-48 Seventieth Road
Forest Hills, NY 11375
718-268-7290

Newsletter; $29 for six issues.

WATER

American Camping Association
5000 State Road 67 N
Martinsville, IN 46151
765-342-8456

CDC National HIV and AIDs Hotline
800-342-2437

For information on filters for *Cryptosporidium*.

Family Campers and RVers
4804 Transit Road, Building 2
Depew, NY 14043
716-668-6242

Water-Filter Certifiers
National Sanitation Foundation
3475 Plymouth Road
Ann Arbor, MI 48106
734-769-8010

Water Quality Association
4151 Naperville Road
Lisle, IL 60532
630-505-0160

Water-Testing Kits
The Clean Water Fund
828-251-0518

Offers home lead-testing kits.

DSK Safer Home Test Kit

Available through twenty-two mail-order catalogs, including:
   Swanson's Health Shopper
   800-437-4148

Enzone
10165 USA Today Way
Miramar, FL 43025
800-448-0535

Frandon Lead Alert Kit
Pace Environs
81 Finchdene Square
Scarborough, Ontario, Canada M1X 1B4
800-359-9000

Solution tests up to a hundred items for lead contamination; $33.45.

John Banta's Healthful Hardware
P.O. Box 3217
Prescott, AZ 86302
520-445-5413

LaMotte Chemical Products Co.
P.O. Box 329
Chestertown, MD 21620
800-344-3100

Kit to test lead in solder; $45.75.

LeadCheck Swabs
HybriVet Systems
P.O. Box 1210
Framingham, MA 01701
800-262-LEAD

One glass vial-swab tests soil, water, and surfaces; eight swabs, $23.45; sixteen swabs, $39.95.

National Testing Laboratories
6555 Wilson Mills Road, Suite 102
Cleveland, OH 44143
800-458-3330
800-426-8378
440-449-2525

Complete line of water-testing kits.

Suburban Water Testing Labs
4600 Kutztown Road
Temple, PA 19560
800-433-6595

Offers a complete line of water-testing services, including home lead-testing kits.

APPENDIX C

Organic Food Sources

Canadian Organic Growers
Box 6408, Station J
Ottawa, Ontario, Canada K2A 3Y6

Publishes *The Directory*, a sourcebook for locating suppliers of organic foods in Canada; about $15 U.S.

Cheese
Brier Run Farm
HC 32, Box 73
Birch River, WV 26610
304-649-2975

Meat
Dakota Mid Meats
136 West Trip
Winner, SD 57580
605-842-3664

Jordan River Farm
6 Shiloh Lane
Huntly, VA 22640
540-636-9388

Certified organic beef and veal.

Lean & Free
RR 3, Box 53
Ackley, IA 50601
800-383-BEEF

Hormone-free beef.

APPENDIX D

Additive-Free Convenience Food

Amy's Kitchen

Arrowhead Mills

Brown rice and peanut butter without herbicides, pesticides, or fertilizers.

Colonel Sanchez

De Bole's

Whole-wheat macaroni and cheese dinner with organically grown flour and cheddar cheese.

Foster Farms

Poultry with pesticide residue elimination policy.

Graindance Pizza

Health Valley

Heart and Soul

Jaclyn's

Legume

Lima

Medallions

Old Chicago Pizza—Lite

Pizsoy

Specialty Grain Company

APPENDIX E

Government Responsibility

Three different governmental agencies are responsible for regulating and monitoring the safety of the U.S. food supply: the U.S. Department of Agriculture (USDA), the Food and Drug Administration (FDA), and the Environmental Protection Agency (EPA).

U.S. DEPARTMENT OF AGRICULTURE (USDA)

The Department of Agriculture monitors the safety of poultry, meat, and eggs and conducts inspections nationwide; it also regulates the use of food and color additives in meat and poultry and inspects eggs and egg products.

Food Safety and Inspection Service (FSIS)

Within the U.S. Department of Agriculture, FSIS is responsible for inspecting meat and poultry products sold in interstate and international trade. These include meat and poultry products imported for sale in this country, which must be produced under inspection systems that meet U.S. standards.

FSIS has the power to recall unsafe or suspicious products after they're on the grocery shelves. Its inspection staff (more than 7,500 poultry and meat inspectors, food technologists, and veterinarians working in more than 7,500 slaughterhouses and processing plants) check meat and poultry for safety.

FSIS also works closely with the food industry on product labels and consumer information. It also monitors facilities and equipment to make sure they meet sanitary requirements.

Finally, FSIS conducts a national consumer education program about proper food handling, including the USDA Meat and Poultry Hotline, which answers questions consumers have about meat and poultry safety.

Agricultural Marketing Service (AMS)

Egg products for sale both in this country and abroad are inspected by the AMS. AMS also conducts USDA's public information campaign about the problem of *Salmonella* bacteria in fresh shell eggs, offering information on proper storage of eggs in both home and institutions.

FOOD AND DRUG ADMINISTRATION (FDA)

The FDA comes under the aegis of the U.S. Department of Health and Human Services and is responsible for ensuring the safety of all food sold in interstate commerce (except meat and poultry). The program is rooted in surprise inspections and sampling of food.

The FDA sets safety limits for drug residues in milk, eggs, meat, and poultry and for some chemical contaminants found in fish. It tests for pesticide residue limits in all food except meat and poultry, develops standards on the quality and safety of food, and regulates food labeling (except for meat, poultry, and alcoholic beverages). The FDA also regulates food additives and veterinary drugs.

ENVIRONMENTAL PROTECTION AGENCY (FDA)

The Environmental Protection Agency is the federal watchdog for all pesticides, regulating the manufacture, labeling, and use of all pesticides, and is responsible for making sure that when used correctly, they don't pose a significant risk to humans or the environment. The EPA also sets tolerance levels for food residues on food sold in the United States, and works with the states to investigate cases of pesticide misuse.

In addition, the EPA sets national drinking water standards for all public water supplies, and provides standards for bottled water modeled on those standards.

NATIONAL MARINE FISHERIES SERVICE

This agency offers a voluntary fee-for-service inspection program for fish products, overseeing about 155 fish processors, brokers, and retail and food service operations. In addition, the service conducts more than four hundred spot inspections each year.

UPDATED SYSTEM

Governmental overview of our food supplies began in 1906 with the passage of the Pure Food and Drug Act and the Meat Inspection Act, designed to make American food as safe as possible. For many years, no new amendments were added to these antiquated laws that used the "poke and sniff" approach—an emphasis on periodic visual inspection of food facilities, supplemented by product testing. Basically, this meant that if meat or poultry didn't look funny or smell bad, it got a stamp of approval.

Unfortunately, *not one* of the deadly microbes now poisoning Americans is visible to the eye or nose: not hepatitis A, not *Salmonella*, not *Listeria*, not *Cryptosporidium*, not *Helicobacter*, and certainly not *E. coli* 0157:H7.

Moreover, for many years the government's primary concern about food poisoning had been *Salmonella*, overlooking many of the other types of bacteria often found in raw food. That narrow concern changed in 1993 when two children died and hundreds more fell ill after eating *E. coli*–tainted hamburger in a fast-food restaurant in Seattle. The incident set off a furor throughout the country, as consumer safety groups urged the government to beef up its meat inspection system.

HACCP

In January 1998, the government implemented a new meat and poultry inspection system called the Hazard Analysis and Critical Control Points (HACCP) involving the 312 largest meat and poultry plants in the United States. These plants account for about 75 percent of all meat and poultry slaughtered in the country.

HACCP addresses the problem of food-borne illness by focusing more attention on the prevention and reduction of microbes on raw products that can cause illness. It also clarifies the roles played by government and industry in protecting the nation's food sources.

The HACCP approach focuses on prevention, using microbiological testings directly targeted at reducing harmful bacteria. It

- requires all meat and poultry plants to develop a system of preventive controls to improve the safety of their products
- sets standards for reducing *Salmonella* bacteria that must be met by slaughterhouses and plants producing raw ground products
- requires all plants to develop written standard operating procedures for sanitation
- tests for *E. coli* contamination

The new system has replaced the old "poke and sniff" approach that had not changed for the previous ninety years, and had been widely criticized as too little, too late.

Under the new system, each plant operates under a HACCP plan designed to prevent contamination of meat or poultry. USDA's FSIS inspectors collect samples to ensure that plants are reducing and controlling the amount of meat or poultry that is contaminated with bacteria. This new approach marks the first time the USDA has required plants to reduce bacterial contamination of raw meat and poultry.

Each plant designs its own plan to meet the USDA food safety guidelines. Basically, each plant must identify all the hazards by which contamination could occur, and then establish critical control points at which they prevent contamination. After the plant sets up the plan, it keeps written records that verify that the system is being followed.

Inspectors will still visually inspect carcasses, document food safety violations, verify a plant's compliance with the HACCP plan, and take direct action when necessary to intercept contaminated meat.

Since the first phase of the plan went into effect in January 1997, the FSIS has shut down twenty plants for failing to meet new standards (compared to the six plants the FSIS shut down in 1996). And through August 1998, the FDA's Center for Food Safety has inspected more than 2,000 seafood processors for HACCP regulations.

Already HACCP has made a difference in food safety. In September 1998, the government reported that *Salmonella* contamination in broiler chickens had been cut in half as a result of the new food-safety system.

For More Information

Information on food-borne disease outbreaks
can be obtained at: Public Inquiries, Centers for
Disease Control and Prevention, 1600 Clifton
Road, Atlanta, GA 30333.

DIET FOR
A POISONED PLANET

How to Choose Safe Foods
for You and Your Family

by David Steinman

Here is your guide to selecting, preparing, and serving the most life enhancing foods available in any supermarket today. Food and water safety expert David Steinman provides you with

- information on which food brands are best;

- reporting on which agricultural regions produce the safest foods;

- scores of tips on how to prepare foods most healthfully;

- a detailed program to eliminate toxins from your body and your home;

- reviews and ratings for hundreds of foods.

Tenth Anniversary Edition!
Updated to include the latest information on new dietary
systems, low-fat eating, food combining,
and alternate medicine

FOOD AND HEALING

by Annemarie Colbin

Drawing on an impressive range of thinking, from Eastern philosophy to contemporary medical journals, Annemarie Colbin argues passionately that we must take responsibility for our own health and rely less on modern medicine, which—even now—seems to focus on trying to cure rather than prevent illness. She includes information on the crucial role of diet in preventing illness, how to tailor a diet approach that is right for you, the remarkable healing qualities of specific foods, and how food affects your moods.

Published by Ballantine Books.
Available in bookstores everywhere.

A Complete Home Reference for
More than 350 Medical Problems and Procedures

THE PDR® FAMILY GUIDE ENCYCLOPEDIA OF MEDICAL CARE™

From *The Physicians' Desk Reference®*

In a world of managed care and rushed appointments, patients often need help in obtaining peace of mind regarding their health concerns. This book puts guidance and information at your fingertips. With a comprehensive alphabetical listing of common and unusual ailments that afflict both children and adults—plus a unique index that matches your signs and symptoms to possible conditions—this is a reassuring home health reference you'll turn to again and again.

Published by Ballantine Books.
Available in bookstores everywhere.